Molecular and Cellular Aspects of the Drug Addictions

Avram Goldstein
Editor

Molecular and Cellular Aspects of the Drug Addictions

Springer-Verlag
New York Berlin Heidelberg
London Paris Tokyo

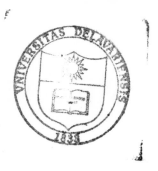

Avram Goldstein, M.D.
Addiction Research Foundation Professor
Department of Pharmacology
School of Medicine
Stanford University
Stanford, California 94305

Library of Congress Cataloging-in-Publication Data
Molecular and cellular aspects of the drug addictions / Avram
  Goldstein, editor.
    p.   cm.
    Based on an all-day symposium held on April 13, 1988.
    Includes bibliographies.
    ISBN 0-387-96827-X (U.S.)
    1. Drug abuse—Physiological aspects—Congresses.
  2. Neurochemistry—Congresses.   3. Drug receptors—Congresses.
  4. Psychopharmacology—Congresses.   I. Goldstein, Avram.
    [DNLM: 1. Substance Dependence—physiopathology—congresses.   WM
  270 M718 1988]
  RC563.2.M64   1989
  615'.78—dc20
  DNLM/DLC
  for Library of Congress   89-10061
                                                   CIP

© 1989 by Springer-Verlag New York Inc.

All rights reserved. No part of this book may be translated or copied in whole or in part without the written permission of the publisher (Springer-Verlag, 175 Fifth Avenue, New York, NY 10010, USA), except for brief excerpts in connection with reviews or scholarly analysis. Use in connection with any form of information storage and retrieval, electronic adaptation, computer software, or by similar or dissimilar methodology now known or hereafter developed is forbidden.
The use of general descriptive names, trade names, trademarks, etc. in this publication, even if the former are not especially identified, is not to be taken as a sign that such names, as understood by the Trade Marks and Merchandise Marks Act, may accordingly be used freely by anyone.
While the advice and information in this book are believed to be true and accurate at the date of going to press, neither the authors nor the editors nor the publisher can accept any legal responsibility for any errors or omissions that may be made. The publisher makes no warranty, express or implied, with respect to the material contained herein.

Typeset by TCSystems, Inc., Shippensburg, Pennsylvania
Printed and bound by Arcata Graphics/Halliday, West Hanover, Massachusetts
Printed in the United States of America.

9 8 7 6 5 4 3 2 1

ISBN 0-387-96827-X Springer-Verlag New York Berlin Heidelberg
ISBN 3-540-96827-X Springer-Verlag Berlin Heidelberg New York

Preface

In 1970 I gave up the chairmanship of the Department of Pharmacology at Stanford University School of Medicine to devote full time to basic and clinical research on problems of drug addiction. In 1971 I developed the method of radioligand binding that led to the important characterization of opioid receptors in several laboratories. The extraordinary specificity of these receptors for morphine and related opiates suggested the likelihood that there were naturally occurring morphine-like molecules in the brain and other tissues. The systematic search for these molecules culminated in 1979 in the discovery, by my group, of the dynorphin peptides—one of the three families of opioid peptides, the first of which (the enkephalin family) had been discovered in Aberdeen, Scotland, in 1975. I also became involved in clinical research on the pharmacologic treatment of heroin addicts, for which I established the first large methadone mainte-nance treatment program in California. My basic and clinical research experience convinced me that an institution encompassing laboratory research, studies on normal human volunteers, and treatment research, under a single roof, could expedite progress in understanding the drug addictions.

That concept was transformed into reality by the founding, in 1974, of the Addiction Research Foundation of Palo Alto, California. The funds for construction of a laboratory were provided by a generous grant from the Drug Abuse Council (a consortium of several foundations), the president of which was Thomas L. Bryant. Strong community support, both in Palo Alto and in San Francisco, came from a number of community leaders, notably Agnes C. Robinson, Martin E. Packard, Brooks Walker, Jr., Jean Kuhn Doyle, Emmett G. Solomon, Henry P. Organ, Herbert Dwight, Jr., Alejandro Zaffaroni, David A. Fasken, David and Lucile Packard, the Honorable Edward C. Scoyen, Leonard Cornell, and Charles G. Schulz.

The Foundation operated independently—it was never affiliated with Stanford—for 14 years. Its research activities were largely funded by the National Institute on Drug Abuse. At the peak of its strength the staff numbered 65, about equally divided between laboratory and clinical research. Leaders of the research teams were Brian M. Cox in the laboratory, Barbara A. Judson in the clinic, and Priscilla Grevert in research on normal human volunteers. The chief administrator was Abbie W. Freiley.

Participating in the Scientific Advisory Board at different times were: Harold Kalant, Floyd E. Bloom, E. Leong Way, Doris H. Clouet, Jack H. Mendelson, Walter M. Booker, William M. Harvey, Jerome H. Jaffe, Murray E. Jarvik, Arnold J. Mandell, and Norman Weiner.

Leo E. Hollister served for many years as chairman of the Human Subjects Committee, which was responsible for reviewing the ethical aspects of all proposed human experiments, and whose membership included numerous medical and lay members of the community.

The Foundation, in its 14 years of existence, had many significant research accomplishments, recorded in more than 200 publications. The major laboratory contributions concerned the dynorphin opioid peptides —their structure, tissue distribution, mode of processing from a large precursor peptide, and their physiologic functions. Human volunteer studies dealt primarily with the natural regulation of pain through the opioid systems, using as a tool the opioid receptor blocker naloxone. Clinical research established optimal dosage regimens for methadone and for the long-acting methadone congener LAAM, developed a practical naloxone test for opiate dependence, worked out effective procedures for drug testing in urine, and advanced our understanding of the principles and efficacy of treating heroin addiction with surrogate opiates or opiate antagonists.

As federal research support faced increasing budgetary constraints, with a resulting instability and unpredictability of research funding by the federal agencies, and with increasing difficulty experienced in fund-raising from the private sector, it became painfully obvious that the dream of a nationally significant multidisciplinary center for addiction research, with its own building and a sufficient endowment to ensure its permanence, was not to be realized. The Board of Directors decided, therefore, to phase out and dissolve the Foundation, but to perpetuate its purpose by transferring all of its cash assets to Stanford University for the purpose of establishing a chair in addiction research in the medical school. The holder of this chair, it was specified, is to have "a demonstrated commitment to teaching and research on the biologic, chemical, and genetic basis of addictive disorders."

All the Foundation's laboratory equipment and supplies were donated to the Department of Physiology of the Beijing Medical University, the People's Republic of China's designated "key" medical university. There Professor J.-S. Han, the department chairman, has carried out important investigations into the functions of the opioid peptides, and has had a long collaborative relationship with the Foundation's scientists. This gift, therefore, will support further research on addiction, pain regulation, and other opioid-related phenomena—research along lines similar to those we followed at Palo Alto.

An all-day symposium was held on April 13, 1988, to mark the dissolution of the Foundation. It was followed by a dinner, at which the Addiction Research Foundation Professorship was presented to Stanford by Martin E. Packard, President of the Foundation, and accepted by Donald Kennedy, President of the University. The symposium speakers were all world-renowned scientists, working either directly on the biological aspects of drug addiction, or on biologic problems germane to the study of the drug addictions. The chapters in this book are based on the lectures presented at the symposium.

Avram Goldstein
Stanford, California
March 3, 1989

Contents

Contributors

Huda Akil, Ph.D., Professor and Director of Research, Department of Psychiatry, Research Scientist, Mental Health Research Institute, Ann Arbor, Michigan 48109-0720, USA

Floyd E. Bloom, M.D., Director, Division of Pre-Clinical Neuroscience and Endocrinology, Research Institute of Scripps Clinic, La Jolla, California 92037, USA

Avram Goldstein, M.D., Addiction Research Foundation, Professor, Department of Pharmacology, School of Medicine, Stanford University, Stanford, California 94305, USA

James P. Herman, Ph.D., Postdoctoral Research Fellow, Mental Health Research Institute, University of Michigan, Ann Arbor, Michigan 48109-0720, USA

A. Herz, M.D., Director, Department of Neuropharmacology, Max Planck Institute for Psychiatry, Planegg-Martinsried, Federal Republic of Germany

Harold Kalant, M.D., Ph.D., Professor, Department of Pharmacology, University of Toronto; Associate Research Director (Biobehavioral Studies), Addiction Research Foundation of Ontario, Toronto, Ontario, Canada

Eric R. Kandel, M.D., University Professor, Center for Neurobiology and Behavior; Senior Investigator, Howard Hughes Medical Institute, Columbia University, College of Physicians and Surgeons, New York, New York 10032, USA

Donald C. Manning, M.D., Ph.D., Department of Neuroscience, Johns Hopkins University School of Medicine, Baltimore, Maryland 21205, USA

Joseph B. Martin, M.D., Ph.D., Julieanne Dorn Professor of Neurology, Harvard Medical School, Boston, Massachusetts 02114, USA

T. S. Shippenberg, Ph.D., Research Assistant, Department of Neuropharmacology, Max Planck Institute for Psychiatry, Planegg-Martinsried, Federal Republic of Germany

Steven A. Siegelbaum, Ph.D., Associate Professor, Department of Pharmacology; Assistant Investigator, Howard Hughes Medical Institute, Columbia University, College of Physicians and Surgeons, New York, New York 10032, USA

Solomon H. Snyder, M.D., Director, Department of Neuroscience, Johns Hopkins Medical School, Baltimore, Maryland 21205, USA

Larry R. Steranka, Ph.D., Nova Pharmaceutical Corporation, Baltimore, Maryland 21224-2788, USA

J. David Sweatt, Ph.D., Associate, Howard Hughes Medical Institute, Columbia University, College of Physicians and Surgeons, New York, New York 10032, USA

Keith A. Trujillo, Ph.D., Postdoctoral Research Fellow, Mental Health Research Institute, University of Michigan, Ann Arbor, Michigan 48109-0720, USA

Andrea Volterra, Ph.D., Associate Research Scientist, Department of Pharmacology; Associate, Howard Hughes Medical Institute, Columbia University, College of Physicians and Surgeons, New York, New York 10032, USA

Stanley J. Watson, Ph.D., M.D., Professor of Psychiatry; Associate Director, Mental Health Research Institute, University of Michigan, Ann Arbor, Michigan 48109, USA

Introduction

Avram Goldstein

Addiction is "a behavioral pattern of drug use, characterized by overwhelming involvement with the use of a drug (compulsive use), the securing of its supply, and a high tendency to relapse after withdrawal" (1).

An expert committee of the World Health Organization (2,3) has for many years struggled with questions of nomenclature in this field. In my opinion, its dogmatic proscribing of the term "addiction" as supposedly imprecise has not been a useful exercise, and the several alternative terms proposed seem to miss the point. "Addiction," as defined above, brings the problem into good focus. It is a behavior, and it concerns the compulsive use of a drug. Thus modern basic research on addiction draws upon the remarkable recent advances in understanding the molecular and cellular bases of two neurobiologic disciplines—psychology and pharmacology.

Discussion of drug addiction in some circles still provokes the fruitless "biology versus psychology" debate—fruitless because we now understand, with ample experimental proofs, that life experiences and environmental stresses alter the neurochemistry of the brain, not only during embryogenesis but also throughout the life span. In short, behavior is a consequence of neurochemistry; psychology is biology. Both the hardware and the software could contribute to addictive behavior, and we need to understand both, in concrete terms, for each addicting drug.

There is obviously no single, simple, cause of addiction. The net contributions of three main factors will determine, at a particular time and place, the incidence and prevalence of addiction to a given drug:

1. Availability of the drug.
2. Individual predisposition to use the drug repeatedly and become addicted.
3. External facilitatory and inhibitory factors such as societal, family, religious, and cultural traditions and attitudes, legal restraints, stressful or tranquil conditions of life, and alternative sources of satisfaction.

Two *consequences* of addiction—tolerance and physical dependence —have been studied extensively at the molecular and cellular levels. Let us first consider *tolerance,* a result of chronic exposure to a drug. There are two kinds. Metabolic tolerance reflects the organism's increased ability to metabolize the drug, so that the drug concentration in contact with the sites of action is reduced. Cellular tolerance represents a decreased sensitivity of the drug-sensitive physiologic systems to a given drug concentration. Both kinds of tolerance have long fascinated pharmacologists (4).

Cellular tolerance is an example of (perhaps only a synonym for) biochemical regulation at the cellular level to maintain homeostasis. Cellular tolerance to opioids (and probably to other addicting drugs) can be selective (5) or can manifest cross-tolerance to unrelated drug families (6). Among the several possible mechanisms is receptor desensitization, which likewise can be homologous (ie, limited to ligands of one receptor type) or heterologous (ie, involving other receptors that converge on the same signal transduction pathway or ion channel) (7).

From a practical standpoint drug tolerance complicates addicts' lives because it requires them to secure ever larger quantities of drug to obtain the desired drug effects. Thus, tolerance as a concomitant of chronic drug use is a relevant subject for study, and it has been studied extensively; but it seems unlikely that research on tolerance will shed light on the molecular and cellular causes of addiction.

Physical dependence represents a physiologic and biochemical adaptation to the presence of an addicting drug so that the organism is seemingly normal while drug concentrations are maintained—concentrations that had produced the characteristic drug effects at the outset. Thus, by definition, physical dependence is accompanied by some degree of tolerance. Removal of the drug unmasks an underlying pathophysiology. This "withdrawal syndrome" is often characterized by effects opposite to the acute pharmacological actions of the drug itself. These disturbances are all relieved dramatically by reestablishing an effective drug concentration.

Although, like tolerance, physical dependence is a consequence, not a precursor of drug addiction, it could nevertheless play a role in initiating repetitive and compulsive drug use after the initial self-administration. The basis for this suggestion is found in two well established facts. First, a measurable small degree of physical dependence is instituted even by the first drug dose (8), so that a withdrawal syndrome (however mild) follows as that initial dose wears off. Second, both animals and humans respond, predictably, to a withdrawal syndrome with intense drug-seeking behavior (9).

The key questions about addiction, in my opinion, have little to do with tolerance or physical dependence. They concern the drug-seeking behavior itself. Why are certain drugs—but not most drugs—sought after and self-administered by people and other animals? What is special about these particular chemical agents? And why is it that even within this restricted set of drugs there is heterogeneity among subjects with respect to self-administration? In some animal strains virtually all individuals self-administer readily, whereas in other strains self-administration is only established with difficulty. And among people, even given equal exposure to an addicting drug, what makes some adopt a pattern of repetitive use and addiction, while others do not? This heterogeneity with respect to predisposition applies to all the addicting drugs; but it is most obvious and unambiguous with licit drugs (e.g., caffeine, nicotine, alcohol), where willingness to engage in antisocial behavior does not becloud the issue.

The addicting drugs belong to five distinct families. As the accompanying table shows, each of these mimics or blocks a particular neurotransmitter in the brain. The barbiturates, benzodiazepines, and ethyl alcohol enhance the actions of γ-aminobutyric acid (GABA), and (except for ethyl alcohol) they have been shown to enhance GABA binding through a specific interaction with the GABA receptor complex (10). Cocaine and the amphetamines block the reuptake of catecholamines at snyapses, thus increasing the local concentration and enhancing the neurotransmitter effects; a putative site of action of cocaine on a

The Addicting Drugs

Drug family	Brain neurotransmitter
Barbiturates Benzodiazepines Ethyl Alcohol	GABA
Cocaine Amphetamines	Catecholamines: Dopamine Norepinephrine Epinephrine (?)
Heroin Morphine Other opiates	Endogenous opioids: Enkephalins Endorphins Dynorphins
Nicotine	Acetylcholine
Caffeine	Adenosine
Phencyclidine (PCP) Cannabinoids (marihuana, THC) LSD Other hallucinogens	?

dopamine transporter was identified recently (11). Morphine (derived from heroin in the body) mimics the actions of one or another endogenous opioid, preferentially binding to and activating the μ type of opioid receptor (12,13). Nicotine, now widely understood to be strongly addictive (14), activates the "nicotinic" type of acetylcholine receptor in brain (15). Caffeine binds specifically, as an antagonist, at an adenosine receptor in brain (16). There is still some uncertainty about the final group in the table, both as to whether they are truly addicting, and as to their biochemical mechanisms and sites of action.

That all the known addicting drugs have a close functional relationship to physiologically important neurotransmitters suggests that in some respect the drug addictions are not so bizarre or pathological or totally foreign to normal processes as one might have thought. In at least a few instances now, the neurochemistry of the addictive drug action has been localized in the brain to so-called "reward pathways" (17–20), some of which are clearly dopaminergic. It appears, in other words, that an addictive drug may stimulate directly a system the physiological role of which is to respond to rewarding (positively reinforcing) life experiences. In this sense addiction seems to represent an artificial activation of a fundamental biologic mechanism for the adaptive regulation of behavior. An interesting question is whether the signals from receptors for different classes of addicting drugs, located on different neurons, converge onto common reward pathways.

The heterogeneity in predisposition, noted above as a feature of all addicting drugs, could well have a strong genetic basis in polymorphisms within the structural and functional elements of the reward pathways. Of great interest, therefore, have been the recent attempts to identify genetic factors in predisposition to drug addiction, thus far primarily predisposition to alcohol addiction (21). The powerful new techniques of molecular biology, such as restriction fragment length polymorphism analysis, are just beginning to be applied here, as in other mental illnesses, and will be used increasingly in drug addiction research (22).

The subject of drug addiction, which arouses great current interest as a societal problem, seems terribly complex and fragmented from the standpoint of scientific understanding at the biologic level. Yet in every complex field of science there comes a time when new modes of thinking and novel experimental (especially reductionist) approaches can stimulate rapid advances, can bring about the kind of scientific revolution described by Kuhn (23). When that happens, new young investigators are attracted, bringing fresh ideas and new techniques from other fields. I believe that such a time may have arrived for the field of drug addiction. At the symposium that was the basis for this book, the lectures offered glimmers of hope for such future developments. It is my hope that the book itself, reaching a wider audience, may further help to stimulate such a transformation.

References

1. Jaffe JH (1985). Drug addiction and drug abuse. In AG Gilman, LS Goodman, TW Rall, F Murad, eds. *The Pharmacological Basis of Therapeutics*, 7th ed. Macmillan, New York.

2. WHO Expert Committee on Drug Dependence, Twentieth Report (1974). World Health Organization Technical Report Series No. 551, Geneva, pp 14–17.

3. Edwards G, Arif A, Hodgson R (1981). Nomenclature and classification of drug- and alcohol-related problems: A WHO Memorandum. *Bull WHO* 59:225–242.

4. Goldstein A, Aronow L, Kalman SM (1974). Drug tolerance and physical dependence. In *Principles of Drug Action*, 2nd ed. Wiley, New York.

5. Schulz R, Wuster M (1984). Molecular mechanisms of opioid tolerance and dependence. *Neuropeptides* 5:3–10.

6. Schulz R, Goldstein A (1973). Morphine tolerance and supersensitivity to 5-hydroxytryptamine in the myenteric plexus of the guinea-pig. *Nature (London)* 244:168–170

7. Sibley DR, Lefkowitz RJ (1985). Molecular mechanisms of receptor desensitization using the β-adrenergic receptor-coupled adenylate cyclase system as a model. *Nature (London)* 317:124–129.

8. Cheney DL, Goldstein A (1971). Tolerance to opioid narcotics, III. Time course and reversibility of physical dependence in mice. *J Pharmacol Exp Ther* 177:309–315

9. Wikler A (1973). Dynamics of drug dependence. Implications of a conditioning theory for research and treatment. *Arch Gen Psychiatry* 28:611–616.

10. Olsen RW, Venter JC, eds (1986). *Benzodiazepine/GABA Receptors and Chloride Channels*. Alan R. Liss, New York. *Receptor Biochemistry and Methodology*, vol 5,

11. Ritz MC, Lamb RJ, Goldberg SR, Kuhar MJ (1987). Cocaine receptors on dopamine transporters are related to self-administration of cocaine. *Science* 237:1219–1223.

12. Udenfriend S, Meienhofer J, eds (1984). *The Peptides*, vol 6, *Opioid Peptides: Biology, Chemistry, and Genetics*. Academic Press, Orlando, FL.

13. Hughes J, Collier HOJ, Rance MJ, Tyers MB, eds (1984). *Opioids: Past, Present and Future*. Taylor & Francis, London.

14. Koop CE (1988). *The Health Consequences of Smoking: Nicotine Addiction*. US Department of Health and Human Services, Washington, DC.

15. Romano C, Goldstein A, Jewell NP (1981). Characterization of the receptor that mediates the nicotine discriminative stimulus. *Psychopharmacologia (Berlin)* 74:310–315.

16. Gould RJ, Murphy KM, Katims JJ, Snyder SH (1984). Caffeine actions and adenosine. *Psychopharmacol Bull* 20:436–440.

17. Wise RA, Bozarth, MA (1985). Brain mechanisms of drug reward and euphoria. *Psychiatr Med* 3:445–460.

18. Vaccarino FJ, Bloom FE, Koob GF (1985). Blockade of nucleus accumbens opiate receptors attenuates intravenous heroin reward in the rat. *Psychopharmacologia (Berlin)* 86:37–42.

19. Olds ME (1979). Hypothalamic substrate for the positive reinforcing properties of morphine in the rat. *Brain Res* 168:351–360.
20. Mucha RF, Herz A (1985). Motivational properties of kappa and mu opioid receptor agonists studies with place and taste preference conditioning. *Psychopharmacologia (Berlin)* 86:274–280.
21. Cloninger CR (1987). Neurogenetic adaptive mechanisms in alcoholism. *Science* 236:410–416.
22. Martin JB (1987). Molecular genetics: applications to the clinical neurosciences. *Science* 238:765–772.
23. Kuhn TS (1970). *The Structure of Scientific Revolutions*, 2nd ed. University of Chicago Press, Chicago.

CHAPTER 1

The Nature of Addiction: An Analysis of the Problem

Harold Kalant

What Is Addiction?

Despite numerous attempts to arrive at standard and universally accepted definitions, the terms "drug abuse," "addiction," and "dependence" continue to be used in different senses by the general public and by experts in different disciplines. Among pharmacologists and physicians there is a widespread tendency to equate addiction with physical dependence, as revealed by the occurrence of a withdrawal syndrome when drug administration is stopped. Yet physical dependence is a consequence of sufficiently prolonged and sufficiently high drug intake, and the fundamental problem is the drug-taking behavior itself. Behavioral scientists tend to equate addiction with dependence (or dependence syndrome), defined as drug-taking behavior that has become preeminent in the user's life, that displaces other goals, that alters social function, and that usually produces tolerance, physical dependence, and other functional or organic disturbances. Physiological alterations in receptor systems, second-messenger systems, and other fundamental components of neurons and other cells may be mechanisms of addiction, or consequences of it, but addiction itself can be defined only in terms of human behavior with respect to drug taking.

The fundamental problems are:

1. Why do humans use psychoactive drugs (and it must be noted that *most* do)?
2. Why do some users become "addicted" (and it must be noted equally that the majority do *not*)?
3. Why do some addicts recover, either spontaneously or as a result of therapeutic intervention of some type, and return either to moderate and problem-free use of drugs or become totally abstinent?

Different disciplines have looked for answers to these questions in different facets of human experience: Sociologists tend to look for answers in the environment and social interactions of human beings; psychiatrists have in the past searched for explanations in terms of internal conflicts or personality disorders, although contemporary biological psychiatrists are more likely to look for answers in terms of changes in neurotransmitter systems; law enforcers try to find explanations in the machinations of drug traffickers; and pharmacologists have tended to seek answers in the pharmacological properties of the drugs themselves, subsumed in such terms as "abuse liability," "dependence potential," and other terms indicative of inherent features of the drug rather than of the user (1). In contrast, in recent years the neurobiologist and the experimental psychologist have looked for answers derived from the concept of reinforcement.

What Is Reinforcement?

In the terminology of operant psychology, developed by Skinner, a reinforcer is any consequence of an individual's action that increases the probability that the individual will repeat that action; the increase in probability is the reinforcement. Therefore, strictly speaking, one can study reinforcement only in an organism that is learning a behavior in order to obtain a reinforcer. In the present context, reinforcement refers to those consequences of self-administration of a drug (the "reinforcer") that increase the probability of taking the drug again. Extensive study of natural reinforcers led to the recognition of two basic types of reinforcement. Positive reinforcement is indicated by the fact that an organism will work to *obtain* a "reward," such as food, water, or access to a sex partner. Negative reinforcement is illustrated by the fact that an organism will work to *remove* or avoid pain, discomfort, or the threat of potential harm. If a behavior results in pain, harm, or discomfort, the behavior is said to be "punished," and therefore the organism learns to *avoid* that behavior because of its "aversive" consequences (2).

Drugs can act as all three—that is, as positive reinforcers, as negative reinforcers, and as punishers. In terms of common human experience, positive reinforcement may contain such elements as the euphoria, increased sociability, and social acceptance that are commonly associated with the moderate social use of alcohol. Negative reinforcement is illustrated by the relief of tension or anxiety that is commonly sought by users of minor tranquilizers, or the relief of boredom that may motivate the use of hallucinogens or volatile solvents. In contrast, punishment is illustrated by such things as the dizziness or nausea that may accompany injudicious use of alcohol, the cough and sense of acute bronchial discomfort that often result from the first experience with cigarettes, or the nausea and disagreeable floating feeling that often characterize the response to opiates in nonaddictive subjects. It is a reasonable assumption that the balance among these three types of consequence determines the degree of probability that the drug taking will be repeated in the future (Figure 1.1).

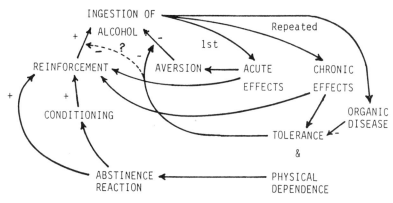

FIGURE 1.1. Schematic representation of consequences of ingestion of ethanol on first exposure and on repeated exposures. + indicates a facilitatory or augmenting effect, − indicates an inhibitory or reducing effect; for example, aversive effects diminish the probability of renewed ingestion of ethanol, tolerance reduces this inhibitory effect, conditioning increases the strength of reinforcement, etc. Reproduced from H. Kalant, *Alcohol and Alcoholism,* Suppl. 1:1–12, 1987; with permission of Pergamon Journals, Ltd., Oxford.

In experimental animals, the positive-reinforcing properties of drugs (properly speaking, the excess of reinforcing properties over aversive properties) are studied by various types of operant self-administration model. The animal is required to learn some motor response, such as pressing on a lever or pecking at an illuminated button to obtain the presentation of a dipper containing a measured volume of drug solution, or to activate a pump so as to inject a measured volume of drug solution via an indwelling cannula ending in a vein, a cerebral ventricle, or some other body location (3–5). The fact that the animal will work to obtain access to the drug is considered, in itself, evidence that the drug has reinforcing properties. By increasing the work load per dose, such as the number of bar presses required, or the complexity of the timing of bar presses required, one can gain a quantitative measure of the strength of those reinforcing properties. The use of such techniques has shown that *most* (but not all) rats, monkeys, dogs, and other laboratory animals readily learn to perform the required task to obtain *some* (but not all) drugs that are used or abused by humans (1,6). Cocaine and opiates are probably the prototypical drugs that have been studied in such models.

Some investigators have assessed the strength of the reinforcing properties of a drug by titrating them against a known amount of punishment incurred by the same response that was required to obtain the drug. For example, Johanson (7) trained rats in an operant chamber equipped with two levers. Pressing on one lever delivered a standard dose of 0.1 mg/kg of cocaine per infusion, whereas pressing on the other lever resulted in delivery of a variable dose of cocaine, with or without a selected intensity of electric foot shock. Typically, the rat would take the standard dose in preference to the same dose, produced by pressure on the other lever, but in combination with foot shock. However, if the second lever resulted in delivery of a higher dose, the animal would take it even when it was accompanied by foot shock. The rats differed considerably with respect to how much the dose had to be raised in order to overcome the punishing effect of the shock. Presumably those rats that required a larger increase found the cocaine less reinforcing than did those animals that were willing to accept shock in return for a smaller increase in dose. It has also been observed repeatedly that if the required work load (i.e., the number of bar presses required to obtain an injection) is raised too much, the animal will stop pressing the lever for drug (8). This observation, together with the finding that the punishing foot shock deterred drug self-administration unless the dose was raised, indicates that the animal was in some manner carrying out a "cost-benefit analysis." Humans clearly do the same, as will be illustrated further below.

Neural Mechanisms of Reinforcement

The analysis of the neural substrates of reinforcement began with the study of intracranial self-stimulation (ICSS), described by Olds and Milner (9). These investigators, and many others subsequently, observed that an animal would readily learn to press a lever in order to deliver a burst of electrical stimuli via electrodes implanted into certain regions of the brain. The most effective sites were the lateral hypothalamus (LH), the median forebrain bundle (MFB), the ventral tegmental area (VTA), and some areas of the prefrontal cortex (10–13). In contrast, similar self-stimulation of certain other areas of the brain resulted in apparently very strong aversive reactions, demonstrated by a sudden and vigorous attempt of the animal to escape from the test situation (14). The first group of sites was interpreted to consist of components of a "reward system" that was suggested to be the brain circuitry responsible for positive reinforcement by natural reinforcers. The second group of sites was considered to constitute the "punishment system" that mediates the aversive effects of noxious stimuli. Fibers in the MFB that are stimulated by "rewarding" ICSS were found to terminate on the A10 dopamine neurons in the VTA, many of which project to dopaminergic terminals in the nucleus accumbens (NACC). Shortly afterwards, it was found that dopamine receptor blockers, such as haloperidol and various D_2 blockers, would interfere with the rat's lever-pressing activity both for natural reinforcers and for ICSS. The result was the postulation of a common reinforcement mechanism for all types of reinforcers, in which inputs from cortex, lateral hypothalamus, and other sites converge on the dopaminergic neurons in the VTA, and the latter, with their projections to the NACC, form the central link (12–14). In keeping with this hypothesis, it has been reported that systemic intraperitoneal (IP) administration of a low dose of ethanol (0.5 g/kg) to freely moving rats led to a large increase in the release of dopamine and its metabolite DOPAC in the NACC, but not in striatum (15). Similar doses increased the spontaneous firing rate of dopamine neurons in A10, the VTA (16). Comparable effects have been reported for morphine (17).

Many psychoactive drugs have been found to facilitate ICSS by lowering the threshold intensity of stimulus required to elicit the ICSS behavior (12,18). The pharmacological category of the drugs does not seem to be critical, as long as the drugs are ones that have reinforcing properties as shown by the self-administration paradigm. For example, both morphine and D-amphetamine cause such lowering of the threshold for ICSS, and the effects of the two drugs are additive (19). Low doses of ethanol, barbiturates, and benzodiazepines have also been found by various investigators to facilitate ICSS at various brain sites (12). Opiates and D-amphetamine are particularly effective when they are injected directly into the VTA. On the other hand, dopamine receptor blockers generally decrease the self-administration of opiates, cocaine, benzodiazepines, and other self-administered drugs (12). From all of this evidence, there has emerged a general consensus that ICSS and self-administered drugs do indeed act upon the same dopaminergic link from the VTA to the NACC.

The picture became complicated somewhat by the discovery that endogenous opioid peptides play a role in the reinforcement process. Various opiates, presumably acting on receptors for endogenous opioids, were found to increase the voluntary consumption of food and water by the rat (20,21). This effect was produced only by the analgesically active isomers and was blocked by naloxone (21). More direct evidence for a role for endogenous opioids in the positive reinforcement process was provided by the observation that the enkephalin analog DADLE caused a dose-dependent increase in food and water intake in the rat, whereas ICI 174,864, and ICI 154,129, which are specific blockers of δ-opioid receptors, decreased the intake of food and water (22). Ingestion of a sweet-tasting liquid was shown to increase the turnover of β-endorphin in the hypothalamus (23), and the administration of naloxone reduced the rat's preference for a sweet solution compared to water (24,25). Therefore, the dopamine theory of reward was modified to include a role for one or more endogenous opioid peptides, possibly as modulators of the activity of dopamine neurons in the VTA. For example, the facilitation by pentobarbital of ICSS in the VTA was reversed by naloxone at a dose (2 mg/kg I.P.) that had no effect by itself, and hence the effect of pentobarbital apparently involved activation of an opioid synapse (26). It has been suggested that an opioid might block the tonic suppression of the dopamine units in the VTA by noradrenergic neurons in the locus ceruleus (27). This function is not a uniquely opioid one because GABA agonists have also been found to increase the spontaneous firing rate of A10 dopamine units, presumably by inhibiting a tonically inhibitory interneuron (28). Such a mechanism might explain how a variety of drugs with quite different pharmacological actions might all activate a common dopaminergic link in the reward mechanism.

Affective Reactions Linked to Reinforcement

At an early stage in the investigation of the reinforcement process, a connection was postulated between reinforcement and certain affective states experienced by the subjects performing reinforced behaviors. In humans acting as experimental subjects, this connection was relatively easy to establish, because when they demonstrated the reinforcing properties of a drug by choosing it in preference to another drug or to a placebo in double-blind tests, they also generally rated the chosen drug higher on a scale of ''liking'' (29). Concurrently, they generally showed higher ratings on subjective rating scales of positive mood (30). Although rats cannot communicate such positive mood verbally, they can nevertheless demonstrate an analogous phenomenon in their behavior. They greet the signaled arrival of a natural reinforcer such as food or water with anticipatory excitement, hyperactivity, sniffing, exploration, and a slight elevation of body temperature, which are generally interpreted as indicators of positive affect (12). These same signs are elicited by signals that the rat has learned to associate with the imminent delivery of drugs shown to be reinforcing in self-administration paradigms. Some investigators have proposed that such increased anticipatory locomotor activity is essential for the process of reinforcement itself (31), although this theory has been challenged by very recent work (32). Nevertheless, it is clear that such hyperactivity accompanies the signaled advent of natural reinforcers, ICSS, opiates, low doses of ethanol, and other reinforcing experiences (13).

The idea that this hyperactivity may be equivalent to the ''liking'' experienced by human drug users is inferred from experiments involving place or taste preference conditioning. If a rat is exposed to a reinforcer in one novel and clearly recognizable environment and to a neutral stimulus in a different but equally recognizable environment, one can then test the animal in an apparatus in which it has free access to both environments and see which it prefers—that is, in which environment it spends more of the total test time (33,34). This technique has shown that the animal reliably prefers the environment in which it has previously received food or access to another rat (35). The interpretation of such findings is that the environment paired with the primary reinforcer comes to serve as a

conditional reinforcer, eliciting the same positive affect that was originally elicited by the reinforcer itself. On the other hand, the animal will
avoid an environment in which it was previously exposed to a punishing
experience such as foot shock. In the same manner, reinforcing or
aversive properties of drugs can be inferred from similar conditioned
preference or aversion to environments previously paired with the drug in
comparison with the drug vehicle (34).

Rats readily acquire a conditioned place avoidance for an environment
previously paired with a known punisher, lithium chloride, and a
preference for an environment previously paired with cocaine (34).
Similarly, the rat prefers the environment previously paired with morphine (Figure 1.2), the extent of the preference being proportional to the
size of the morphine dose (36), and again only the $l(-)$ isomers give rise to
conditioned preferences while the $d(+)$isomers do not (37). Naloxone
blocks the development of a morphine-conditioned place preference (36),
and somewhat larger doses of naloxone alone give rise to a conditioned
place aversion (38,39). The magnitude of this latter effect is dependent on

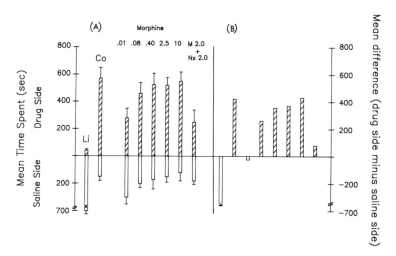

FIGURE 1.2. Conditioned place preferences elicited in rats by pairing one
environment (of a two-environment test apparatus) with saline and the other with
a drug. Drugs shown are (from left) LiCl 60 mg/kg, cocaine 10 mg/kg, morphine
0.01, 0.08, 0.40, 2.5, and 10 mg/kg, and morphine 2 mg/kg + naloxone 2 mg/kg.
Naloxone was injected IP, all other drugs IV. A. Plotted values are the test results
during free access to both environments in the absence of any drug injection.
Values above the line indicate time (in seconds) spent in the previously drug-
paired environment; values below the line indicate time spent in the previously
saline-paired environment. B. Mean preference or aversion for each drug,
expressed as the difference between the time spent on the drug-paired side and the
time spent on the saline-paired side. Values above the line indicate preferences;
value below the line indicates aversion. Drawn from data of Mucha et al (34).

the dose of naloxone. The naloxone-conditioned place aversion probably reflects naloxone blockade of an action of an endogenous opioid in the positive reinforcement system. This explanation is supported by three types of evidence. First, β-endorphin itself has been shown to give rise to a conditioned place preference, which is blocked by naloxone (40). Second, destruction of the arcuate nucleus in the basomedial hypothalamus drastically reduces the amount and turnover of β-endorphin in the brain and at the same time abolishes the place-aversion effect of naloxone (38). Third, chronic exposure to naltrexone from a subcutaneously implanted slow-release pellet increases the ability of previously sub-threshold doses of morphine to elicit conditioned place preference in the rat, presumably as a result of μ-receptor up-regulation (41). Thus the conditioned aversion produced by naloxone probably does not reflect a direct aversive effect of naloxone as much as the removal by naloxone of a tonic reinforcing effect of an endogenous opioid.

Similar conditioning techniques can be used in connection with taste preference or aversion. An animal that experiences for the first time the effects of a drug while it is allowed to drink a liquid flavored with a novel but affectively neutral taste will show in subsequent testing a conditioned preference for that taste versus water if the drug effect was reinforcing, and a conditioned preference for water versus the novel taste if the drug effect was aversive. Although there are some significant differences between the results of testing the same drug by the conditioned place preference and the conditioned taste preference techniques (42), in general the two methods give sufficiently concordant results that they are considered to reflect the same properties of the drugs. In addition, many pharmacological interventions produce similar changes in drug-conditioned behaviors and in self-administration. For example, systemic administration of haloperidol and injection of 6-hydroxydopamine into the NACC were found to block diazepam-induced conditioned place preference (43) just as they had been shown to block drug self-administration (12).

Evidence that Does Not Fit

The evidence reviewed up to this point appeared to indicate a remarkable degree of concordance among the findings obtained by studies of operant drug self-administration, drug enhancement of ICSS, and indirect indicators of the affective and motivational properties of drugs. However, a closer examination indicates many problems in the form of evidence that does not fit the scheme outlined above. For example, whereas De Witte and Bada (44) found facilitation of ICSS in the lateral hypothalamus by ethanol in doses of 0.3 and 0.6 g/kg IP, Schaefer et al (45) found a dose-dependent depression of ICSS and of locomotor activity over a similar dose range. Moreover, it is not totally certain that ICSS itself is really the equivalent of reinforcement by natural reinforcers. As noted earlier, there is a "punishment system" in the brain, functionally opposite to the "reward system." Sites such as the dorsal periaqueductal gray matter, the medial hypothalamus, and the reticular formation make up part of the punishment system. If the experimenter applies an electrical stimulus in those areas to the conscious rat, the rat makes a very strong escape response. Nevertheless, mice have been shown to self-stimulate those same regions through implanted electrodes in a manner comparable to self-stimulation in the NACC or MFB (14). This result is in some respects comparable to the observation that rats will self-administer foot shock, which is aversive when administered by the experimenter (46). This type of evidence creates some degree of uncertainty about the assumption that ICSS reflects exclusively positive reinforcement or the equivalent of the human "liking."

Another problem is that the effect of dopamine receptor blockers on ICSS may not be equivalent to loss of reinforcement. The "rewarding efficacy" of ICSS has been estimated in terms of a shift in the curve relating the bar-pressing rate to the current strength (in microamperes) or pulse frequency of the ICSS stimuli. Under the influence of pimozide or other neuroleptics, this curve shows a lateral shift of at most 0.3 log units—ie, a 50% reduction in reward efficacy. In contrast, manipulation of the current strength can shift the rate-frequency function by one whole log unit or more, and intracerebroventricular (ICV) injection of atropine can shift it as much as 0.6 log units (47). The shallow slope of the curve under the influence of neuroleptics and the sudden cutoff of all responding above a certain dose have been interpreted as evidence that neuroleptics do not block the reward process; rather, they block either the memory of having received the reward or the ability to initiate a complex response necessary to obtain it. This hypothesis is consistent with a recent observation that haloperidol and flupenthixol suppress bar pressing by the rat for water reinforcement more than they impair simple licking of the spout of a water bottle (48). Moreover, increasing the number of bar presses required to obtain each water reinforcement (which, as noted above, can overcome the reinforcing efficacy of natural reinforcers) did not increase the inhibitory effect of haloperidol on bar pressing for water. This fact also argues against a reduction of the reinforcing property of water by haloperidol and is more consistent with the idea that initiation of the response is impaired.

One of the most puzzling problems is that ethanol, one of the psychoactive drugs most widely used by humans, has been shown repeatedly to give rise to conditioned place avoidance rather than conditioned place preference, regardless of whether the alcohol is given intravenously, by intragastric administration, or by intraperitoneal injection (49–51). The same is true of pentobarbital, which gives rise to progressively greater degrees of conditioned place aversion as progressively larger doses are used in the training (52). Benzodiazepines, which are also widely used and abused by humans, produce only weak and inconsistent conditioned place preference (53) and are not as readily self-administered as barbiturates (54). The findings, which suggest a marked preponderance of aversive over reinforcing effects of ethanol, are supported by other evidence such as the observations that rats will actively work to avoid injections of ethanol (55) and display a conditioned place aversion to an environment in which they have previously consumed alcohol solutions voluntarily (56). Nevertheless, rats will readily learn to perform an operant task to gain access to ethanol (57,58), and under these circumstances will consume it orally in large amounts and at concentrations as high as 16% or 32% w/v, which are ordinarily highly aversive in simple two-bottle-choice drinking tests. Therefore it is not at all clear that one can necessarily equate operant reinforcement with conditioned place preference under all circumstances.

Since ethanol is readily oxidized by most mammals and many other species, to yield 7 kcal/g of ethanol, there has long been a debate in the alcohol research literature as to whether ethanol is consumed by laboratory rats for its pharmacological reinforcing effects or as a food analogous to starch or fat. One fact that appeared to support the argument that it is taken as a food is that restriction of the solid food ration leads to a large increase in ethanol consumption, and restoration of *ad libitum* feeding causes the ethanol intake to fall again (59). However, food restriction causes exactly the same effect on voluntary ingestion of opiates, cocaine, barbiturates, and other drugs that make no significant caloric contribution (8,60). Therefore food deprivation must in some way enhance the effectiveness of other reinforcers, although this concept has not yet been adequately explained.

Another major problem is that there is no real agreement on the dopaminergic link from the VTA to the NACC as the common basis of positive reinforcement by ICSS or by different drugs, or even by cocaine, the best-studied one. There is disagreement as to whether reinforcement is mediated by D_1 receptors (11) or D_2 (61–63) receptors. Many types of evidence point to the possibility that other pathways are associated with reinforcement. For example, opiates can give rise to conditioned place preference after direct injection into various other sites in the brain, including the caudate, the lateral hypothalamus, and the periaqueductal gray (36). Conversely, the injection of opiate receptor blockers at sites other than the VTA and the NACC has also yielded evidence for the participation of these other sites in the reinforcement process. Methylnaltrexone, a quarternary derivative of naltrexone, is an obligatory cation and therefore does not diffuse readily across cell membranes. When injected into specific brain sites in small volumes, it tends to remain at those sites for a considerable period of time. Local microinjections of methylnaltrexone into NACC, periaqueductal gray, and lateral hypothalamus are all able to raise the rate of responding for intravenous heroin, a result that is typical of the effect of a decrease in reinforcement (64,65). The subject appears to be increasing the response rate in an effort to overcome the diminished reinforcing efficacy of the drug. However, the injection of methylnaltrexone into the medial prefrontal cortex did not increase the rate of responding for intravenous heroin (64). In contrast, it has been reported that rats will self-inject cocaine directly into the medial prefrontal cortex, but not into the NACC or the VTA. Moreover, sulpiride (a D_2 dopamine receptor blocker) did not affect the baseline response rate by itself, but significantly decreased the response rate for self-injection of cocaine directly into the medial prefrontal cortex (61,62).

Several other lines of evidence point to the probability of separate neural systems mediating the reinforcing effects of heroin and of cocaine. For example, intraperitoneal injection of naltrexone in doses ranging from 0.1 to 10 mg/kg, or injection of methylnaltrexone (0.1–3 μg) into the periaqueductal gray, produced dose-dependent increases in the rate of bar pressing for self-administration of intravenous heroin, as would be predicted for the effects of partial loss of reinforcing efficacy, but similar administration of these opioid receptor blockers did not affect the rate of self-administration of cocaine (65,66). In contrast, α-flupenthixol produced a dose-dependent increase in the response rate for cocaine but did not affect the rates for heroin (66). Similarly, destruction of the dopamine terminals by direct injection of 6-hydroxydopamine into the NACC produced a time-dependent decrease or extinction of cocaine self-administration, whereas self-administration of heroin was reduced only initially, but then recovered almost to the prelesion levels by five or six sessions after the production of the lesion (67). Rats treated with dopamine receptor blockers still demonstrate morphine-conditioned place preference (68). Lesions produced by microinjections of 6-hydroxydopamine into the VTA or NACC of rats caused hypersensitivity to the behavioral effects of an enkephalin derivative acting in NACC (69). Since such dopamine neuron lesions do not produce up-regulation of opioid receptors in NACC, this finding was interpreted as evidence that dopaminergic and enkephalinergic systems function in parallel rather than in series.

All of these lines of evidence point to the possible existence of separate parallel neural systems that mediate the reinforcing effects of cocaine and heroin, and possibly of other drugs as well. In addition, they point to the participation in the reinforcement process of a variety of sites and pathways in the brain. Further evidence indicates that a number of other neurotransmitters apart from dopamine play important roles in reinforcement. For example, electrical stimulation of the VTA gives rise to discriminative stimuli, linked to reinforcement, which can be facilitated by amphetamine and blocked by haloperidol when the stimulation is carried out in extended trials at low frequency (70), but is enhanced by physostigmine when the stimulation is carried out in more frequent trials of short duration (71). These findings implicate dopamine and acetylcholine in different aspects of the reward system.

The observation noted earlier, that atropine produces a greater lateral displacement of the ICSS reward efficacy curve than haloperidol does (47), also suggests that acetylcholine acting at central muscarinic receptors is involved in some way. Moreover, rats that were actively self-injecting morphine showed large changes in the turnover of norepinephrine, serotonin, aspartate, and γ-aminobutyric acid in many areas of the brain, in comparison to the turnovers observed in "yoked" rats—that is, rats receiving passively the same doses of morphine at the same times as the self-administered doses taken by the active rats (72). The fact that the rats carrying out the self-injection showed differences from those receiving the same injections passively is good evidence that the observed changes were not due to the actions of morphine itself. The observed changes in neurotransmitter turnover are not necessarily related directly to the reinforcement process, because they may be associated with various components of the motor or sensory pathways associated with bar-pressing behavior. Nevertheless, the findings point to a number of specific areas and specific transmitters, the association of which with the reinforcement process clearly requires further exploration.

Aspects of Dependence Unexplained by Current Reinforcement Models

It is important to recognize that these various approaches to the study of reinforcement leave unanswered a great many very important questions relating both to drug use and to drug dependence or addiction. A few of these major questions are pointed out below.

Negative Reinforcement

All of the studies described above deal only with exploration of the nature of positive reinforcement by natural reinforcers, ICSS, or psychoactive drugs. Yet negative reinforcement is widely believed to play an important role in psychoactive drug use and in the continuation of dependence on such drugs. For example, in experiments with human subjects, the choice of diazepam in preference to placebo was accompanied mainly by feelings of sedation and decreased anxiety rather than euphoria or other positive affect (30). Among alcoholics and opiate addicts, continued use of the drug is often attributed, at least in part, to its ability to relieve unpleasant withdrawal symptoms (12,13). The profound depression that follows sudden cessation of prolonged high-dose use of cocaine or amphetamine is frequently pointed to as the cause of relapse, renewed drug taking being interpreted as self-therapy for the alleviation of the depression (73–75). All of these examples of negative reinforcement are still unexplained in terms of neural mechanisms (12). Rats in which all forebrain structures except the hypothalamus had been removed were still able to learn to avoid a spontaneous "uphill" orienting response when this behavior was punished by administration of shock to the tail. Moreover, rats that had learned the avoidance response before removal of the forebrain structures were still able to perform the avoidance correctly after recovery from the surgery (76). These findings indicate that both the acquisition and the storage of the learned avoidance—and therefore, by implication, the negative reinforcement—took place at levels below the forebrain. This site apears to be in striking contrast to the preponderantly forebrain location of the positive reinforcement pathways.

Individual Differences

The proposed model of positive reinforcement described above does not take into account the very clear interindividual differences observed in both humans and experimental animals. It does not include any explanation of why the same drug can be reinforcing in some subjects and aversive in others or of why reinforcement can be mild in one case and apparently strong enough to lead to addiction in another. For example, human subjects who consistently chose amphetamine over placebo in double-blind experiments reported that it increased their positive mood and produced euphoria, whereas those who consistently chose the placebo reported that amphetamine increased their anxiety level and lowered their positive mood (30).

In recent years a great deal of interest has centered on possible genetic differences, principally in relation to the predisposition to alcoholism. A number of excellent detailed reviews of this topic have appeared in the past few years, and the interested reader is referred to them for a full discussion of the subject (77–79). Only a few points will be recapitulated here.

It has long been known that alcoholism tends to run in families. Studies of twins, half-siblings, and individuals adopted very early in infancy (before they could possibly have learned anything from their biological parents) have all confirmed the probable existence of a genetic factor associated with a threefold to fourfold increase in the risk of alcoholism. Family pedigree studies have shown that the degree of additional risk is proportional to the number of generations showing positive family history for alcoholism on both sides of the family (80). However, it has never been established clearly exactly what is inherited. It is evident that the children of alcoholics do not inherit a gene for alcoholism itself, but rather for some trait that increases the degree of probability that they may become alcoholic.

Several investigators have observed that the sons of alcoholic biological fathers are less affected by a given dose of ethanol than the sons of nonalcoholic fathers are, in such measures as subjective ratings of intoxication, standing ataxia in the Romberg test (81), or changes in specific components of electroencephalographic recordings (82). However, the physiological measures that have been used in these studies are signs of intoxication rather than of reward. Therefore, these findings point only to possible reasons why the sons of alcoholics *can* drink more and not why they *do*. Genetically decreased sensitivity to these effects might result in a decreased "cost-benefit" ratio for alcohol in those individuals, but it does not shed any light on the nature of the "reward" that motivates greater drinking in alcoholics. The finding of differences in event-related potentials in sons of alcoholics, in the complete absence of any exposure to alcohol (83), are of greater interest for this reason.

Animal studies lend themselves better for a more detailed and specific analysis of the genetic factors involved in alcohol drinking or alcohol preference. The level of alcohol consumption in a free choice of alcohol solution versus water is normally distributed in a large randomly chosen population of rats. By the selective mating of high drinkers with high drinkers and low with low, it has been possible to develop two strains—a high-drinking and a low-drinking strain—from the starting population (84). Three such genetic selections have now been carried on over many generations, each giving rise to two stable lines: the UChA and UChB lines (85), the AA and ANA lines (86), and the P and NP lines (87). The P and NP selection is particularly striking, in that the P rats voluntarily consume large enough quantities of alcohol every day to show high blood alcohol levels, intoxication, development of tolerance, and physical dependence (87). It has not yet been established whether they will consume enough over a sufficiently long time to produce some of the characteristic organic complications of alcoholism, but this topic is undoubtedly under current investigation.

Apart from these strains specifically selected for differences in alcohol consumption, there are many inbred mouse strains selected for other purposes, such as susceptibility to cancer transplant, which have also been found to differ with respect to voluntary consumption of ethanol (88). These differences are currently being exploited in molecular genetic studies aimed at identifying the gene responsible for the differences in drinking behavior. A recent report (89) describes the identification of a specific protein polymorphism correlated with the strain differences in voluntary intake of alcohol, thereby permitting the identification of a single gene accounting for most of the variance in alcohol intake. In similar studies of human families whose pedigrees permit the tracing of genetic susceptibility to alcoholism, it should be possible to apply the same molecular genetic techniques to lymphocytes or other cells in a search for a gene or genes predisposing to alcoholism in humans.

Other genetic selection studies in rats have isolated two lines, the LC2-Hi and LC2-Lo strains, characterized by high and low rates, respectively, of ICSS in the lateral hypothalamus. These lines showed a conditioned place preference and conditioned place aversion, respectively, for environments previously paired with administration of morphine or heroin. Conversely, the LC2-Hi strain showed a much greater conditioned place aversion to naloxone than did the LC2-Lo line (90). These findings raise a similar possibility for molecular genetic identification of a specific gene responsible for differences in reinforcement by opiates. There is no *a priori* reason why a similar approach should not be applied to the analysis of genetic factors determining reinforcement by other types of drug.

A considerable degree of caution is required, however, with respect to the interpretation of such studies. In the case of the gene controlling the intake of ethanol by mice, it is not clear what the gene actually controls for. Among the possibilities that must be considered in rodents are relative sensitivity to the aversive taste of ethanol, differences in the ability to utilize calories derived from the metabolism of ethanol, differences in the ability to develop acute and/or chronic tolerance to the aversive effects of ethanol (87,88), and differences in the degree of reinforcement obtained from ethanol (91). None of these possibilities has yet been explored specifically. P rats are known to differ from NP not only with respect to the level of voluntary consumption of ethanol, but also in initial sensitivity to the intoxicating effects and the ability to develop acute (ie, within-session) tolerance (87). Yet gene differences are typically extremely selective, determining polymorphisms in a single protein, and would therefore be expected to produce quite selective differences in drug responses. For example, mice selected genetically for sensitivity or resistance to ethanol withdrawal seizures did not differ with respect to sensitivity to various signs of acute intoxication, ethanol metabolism, or ability to acquire ethanol tolerance (92). Therefore it is not clear which of the possibilities mentioned above is primary in the differentiation of the P and NP rats or whether there are multiple genetic differences.

This question is particularly important because recent human studies have shown that there are at least two quite different patterns of genetic influence with respect to alcoholism or problem drinking (93). One identified pattern, which has the much stronger genetic component, is that of the predominantly male pattern of alcoholism characterized by early onset, rapid progression of the behavior disorder, high frequency of impulsive and antisocial behavior, and poor response to treatment. The other pattern, characterized by later onset, slower progression, milder course, better treatment response, and much higher dependence on evironmental or situational contributing factors, is much more frequently encountered among human alcoholics but has a lower genetic component.

Thus it is suggested that more than one gene must be involved in human alcoholism and also that the gene or genes affect the relative risk of becoming alcoholic but are not absolute determinants.

Similarly, even in the genetically selected animal strains, the gene is not the absolute controller of voluntary alcohol intake. For example, work in our own laboratories (Beardsley, Kalant, Woodworth, and Stiglick, manuscript in preparation) has shown that operant training of mildly food-restricted rats can induce the ANA strain to increase its alcohol consumption almost to the same level as that shown initially by the alcohol-preferring AA strain. In this paradigm, in which the rats can press separate levers to obtain either alcohol or water that are concurrently available, the ANA rats will work to obtain substantial amounts of even 32% ethanol, although they never consume as much as the AA rats at any given concentration.

It is clear that the genetic factor, though important, interacts with environmental and behavioral factors in determining the extent to which a genetic risk is converted into a reality of alcohol drinking or alcoholism.

Previous Individual History

Another phenomenon that current models of drug reinforcement do not explain is the extent to which the individual's previous history affects the apparent degree of reinforcement by drugs. For example, monkeys that had been previously trained to self-administer codeine and were then tested with other opiates took more of these other opiates than animals that had been previously trained on cocaine and were then transferred to the same drugs (94). Similarly, monkeys trained on pentobarbital established benzodiazepine self-administration more easily than monkeys trained on cocaine (54). This finding raises the possibility that subjective discriminative stimuli generated by the training drug may influence what the animal experiences as ''reward'' or ''aversion.''

Some support for this idea is provided by a number of observations indicating that the subjective discriminative stimuli generated by one drug can become the appropriate or necessary cues for the manifestation of conditioned taste aversion or preference generated by a second drug. For example, the presence or absence of naloxone could be used as cues to control the appearance of a conditioned taste aversion to saccharin followed by an emetic agent (95). Similar effects have been reported for morphine (96), phencyclidine (97), and amphetamine and pentobarbital (98). A similar explanation might account for the observation that rats that had been made dependent on morphine and then withdrawn for 1 to 4 months showed a much greater hyperactivity response to low doses of morphine or methadone, but not of pentazocine, than controls did (99). Hyperactivity, as noted above, is a typical response to reinforcers, and the increased response in previously dependent animals might reflect motivational effects via μ-receptors (but not κ-receptors) as a conditioned response to discriminative stimuli produced by low doses of μ-agonists.

Another important factor related to the individual's past drug history is tolerance. Tolerance to a wide variety of aversive effects of ethanol, opiates, cannabis, amphetamine, and other drugs has been very clearly demonstrated, as shown by a voluminous literature on the subject (100–103). It is commonly held that this tolerance to aversive effects of a drug *permits* the ingestion of much larger amounts of the drug before the further self-administration is stopped by the appearance of toxic effects. It is much less clear, however, that tolerance can occur to the positive reinforcing effects of a drug and thus *require* the ingestion of larger amounts in order to achieve the same "reward" that was initially achieved with smaller doses. Most investigations have failed to reveal any tolerance to the positive reinforcing effects of psychoactive drugs (104). However, whereas acute administration of D-amphetamine to the rat reduces the stimulus threshold intensity necessary to sustain ICSS behavior, chronic administration produced a clear increase in the stimulus threshold intensity that was evident when the drug was stopped; hence continued administration of amphetamine was needed to bring the threshold back down to the normal baseline (105,106). This finding was interpreted as evidence for both tolerance to and physical dependence on amphetamine. This interpretation seems eminently reasonable because the pattern of changes is analogous to the acute elevation of electroshock seizure threshold by ethanol, the overshoot to a subnormal seizure threshold during the withdrawal period after chronic ethanol administration, and the normalization of threshold by the reinitiation of ethanol administration (107). However, this example is an isolated one, and much more thorough study is required to establish whether tolerance does or does not occur to the reinforcing effects of other drugs in other test paradigms.

Interaction with Socioeconomic Factors

Another very important phenomenon that cannot yet be explained by any purely neurobiological model of drug reinforcement is the interaction between drug "reward" and social and economic influences as determinants of the levels of drug intake. For example, epidemiological studies have revealed quite different patterns of drug preference among comparable groups of addicts in Bangkok, Jakarta, Islamabad, and other centers (108). It seems extremely improbable that human biology can differ sufficiently from country to country to account for the preference for opium in one location, cannabis in another, and volatile solvents in a third. It seems much more reasonable to attribute these differences to local habit, availability, and peer group fads and fashions.

The price of alcohol, expressed in relation to current disposable income, has been shown to be a major determinant of variation in levels of alcohol consumption within the same population over time (Figure 1.3), not only in the general population of social drinkers but also in the subpopulation of alcoholics (109–111). For example, the death rate from alcoholic cirrhosis of the liver has been shown to be inversely related to the price of alcohol (112). This price elasticity of alcohol consumption, in both light and very heavy drinkers, has been demonstrated experimentally (113). In a long-term experiment in a residential research ward, involving a group of social drinkers and a group of alcoholics, the subjects performed work for which they were paid with tokens that could be used to purchase various amenities including alcohol, or which could be saved up and redeemed for a very substantial amount of money at the end of the experiment. The alcoholics as a group purchased many more drinks during the observation period than the social drinkers did, but within each group a subgroup that had access to the alcohol at half price for several hours a day (''happy hour'') drank twice as much as the other subgroup, which did not have the benefit of the price reduction. Similarly, current observations suggest that the level of consumption of cocaine in the North American population is markedly affected by the price. A survey of cocaine users indicated that the upper income group used an average of 15 grams per week, while the middle income group used 8.2 g/wk (114). The

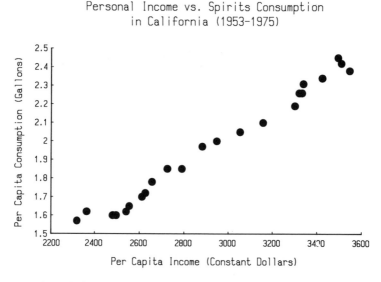

FIGURE 1.3. Relation between per capita annual personal income in constant (deflated) dollars and per capita consumption of distilled spirits (gallons per year) in the state of California, 1952–1975. Plotted values are not in exact chronological sequence. Similar results were obtained for beer and for California wine. Drawn from data of Bunce (110).

introduction of the less purified and therefore cheaper free-base form known as "crack" is reported to be associated with a large increase in the amount of cocaine use by high school students and others with limited amounts of money to spend on nonessentials (115).

Two substances that are widely used and socially accepted in most countries of the world, nicotine and caffeine, are also recognized as being potentially addictive. The great difficulty experienced by smokers in attempting to stop cigarette smoking is fully consistent with many experimental demonstrations of the strong reinforcing properties of nicotine in humans and experimental animals (116), and a nicotine withdrawal syndrome has recently been described in smokers randomly assigned to either total cessation of smoking, 50% reduction, or substitution of low-nicotine cigarettes (117). Reinforcing properties of caffeine, and a caffeine withdrawal syndrome in human subjects, have also been described (118,119). The use of caffeine in North America has not changed markedly in many years, but the prevalence of daily cigarette smoking, most of which can probably be described as dependent use, has diminished sharply in recent years. Canadian survey data have shown a remarkable change in the pattern of distribution of daily smoking, as well as in the absolute level (120). Older age cohorts consistently showed a much higher prevalence of daily smoking among males than among females, regardless of the level of education. The youngest cohort in the study, however, shows that the male-female difference has almost disappeared, and that for both sexes those with secondary school education or less are much more likely to be daily smokers than those with at least some university or postsecondary education (Figure 1.4). It is impossible to explain this change in the sex difference by any change in the biology of reinforcement by nicotine, so the recent change in smoking patterns must reflect such factors as the greater social independence of women, the increasing concern with healthy life-style, and the increasing effects of education on public awareness of the health hazards of smoking.

Apart from the social and economic influences mentioned above, as-yet-unexplained factors have also been held to be responsible for long-term fluctuations in levels of alcohol consumption in many countries (121). Official records from various sources have indicated a gradual fall in mean per capita consumption of alcohol in most countries of northern Europe and North America, beginning in the middle of the nineteenth century and continuing until the late 1930s, followed by a steady postwar rise to a peak in the late 1970s or early 1980s. Superimposed minor year-to-year fluctuations were randomly distributed around the main trend line. In contrast, in the wine-producing countries of Europe, especially France and Italy, the mean per capita consumption remained relatively constant over this long period of observation. These long-term trends appear to be independent of any recognizable changes in price,

PREVALENCE OF DAILY CIGARETTE SMOKING IN CANADA

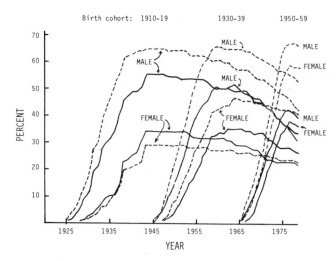

FIGURE 1.4. Prevalance of daily cigarette smoking among three birth cohorts in Canada during the years 1925–1977. Cohorts were those born in 1910–1919, 1930–1939, and 1950–1959. Separate curves are drawn for males and females, and for those with only high school education or less (————) and those with some university or other postsecondary education (————). Ordinate: percent of each group who were daily smokers during the year shown on the abscissa. Redrawn from Ferrence (120), with permission of the author.

legal status, or other recognizable policy factors, and have been attributed to changes in the drinking culture and social attitudes in the affected countries, through the operation of social network mechanisms that affect values and practices at the local level (121). It is self-evident that such fluctuations cannot be attributable to any changes in the reinforcing or other properties of the drugs themselves.

Conclusion

The very large body of evidence on which this brief review has been based indicates clearly that drugs have demonstrable reinforcing properties; however, despite much detailed analysis of the neurobiological basis of reinforcement, the mechanism is not yet clearly known. Moreover, the modification of reinforcing or aversive properties of drugs within the same individuals, as a result of situational or experiential factors, has been largely unstudied. The role of tolerance to aversive effects of drugs has been well established, but the possibility of tolerance to the reinforcing effects has been only minimally explored. Large areas of human experience about drug use and addiction, including the numerous social and economic factors mentioned above, do not yet have parallels in the laboratory models used to study the biological basis of addiction in experimental animals. No satisfactory explanation has yet been provided as to how the reinforcing properties of drugs, which determine at least in part the probability of their being used by humans, can account for the fact that most users are not addicted and only a small and variable fraction are.

It is therefore evident, from all of these gaps in our present knowledge, that the biological basis of addiction has not yet been satisfactorily explained. Any hope for a specific preventive or therapeutic intervention based on neurobiological knowledge is unlikely to be fulfilled until some of these major gaps in our knowledge have been bridged. This fact, rather than discouraging research, should constitute one of the strong arguments for continued experimental, clinical, and epidemiological analysis of the nature of addiction.

Acknowledgments. The author is indebted to R.F. Mucha, W.A. Corrigall, and other colleagues for valuable discussions of the work on reinforcement mechanisms; to Roberta Ferrence for making available her data on smoking, before publication of her Ph.D. dissertation; to John Mihic for preparation of some of the figures; and to Valdemira Cabral for skillful preparation of the manuscript.

References

1. Brady JV, Lukas SE (1984). *Testing Drugs for Physical Dependence Potential and Abuse Liability.* NIDA Research Monograph 52. US Department of Health and Human Services, Washington, DC.
2. Deese J, Hulse SH (1967). *The Psychology of Learning,* 3rd ed. McGraw-Hill, New York, pp 24–27.
3. Weeks JR (1962). Experimental morphine addiction: Method for automatic intravenous injections in unrestrained rats. *Science* 138:143–144.
4. Deneau G, Yanagita T, Seevers MH (1969). Self-administration of psychoactive substances by the monkey. *Psychopharmacology* 16:30–48.
5. Schuster CR, Johanson CE (1974). The use of animal models for the study of drug abuse. In RJ Gibbins, Y Israel, H Kalant, RE Popham, W Schmidt, RG Smart, eds. *Research Advances in Alcohol and Drug Problems,* vol. 1. Wiley-Biomedical, New York, pp 1–31.
6. Thompson T, Unna KR, eds (1977). *Predicting Dependence Liability of Stimulant and Depressant Drugs.* University Park Press, Baltimore.
7. Johanson CE (1977). The effects of electric shock on responding maintained by cocaine injections in a choice procedure in the rhesus monkey. *Psychopharmacology* 53:277–282.
8. Meisch RA (1987). Factors controlling drug reinforced behavior. *Pharmacol Biochem Behav* 27:367–371.

9. Olds J, Milner P (1954). Positive reinforcement produced by electrical stimulation of septal area and other regions of rat brain. *J Comp Physiol Psychol* 47:419–427.

10. Routtenberg A (1981). Drugs of abuse and the endogenous reinforcement system: The resistance of intracranial self-stimulation behavior to the inebriating effects of ethanol. *Ann NY Acad Sci* 362:60–66.

11. Mora F, Ferrer JMR (1986). Neurotransmitters, pathways and circuits as the neural substrates of self-stimulation of the prefrontal cortex: Facts and speculations. *Behav Brain Res* 22:127–140.

12. Wise RA (1987). The role of reward pathways in the development of drug dependence. *Pharmacol Ther* 35:227–263.

13. Wise RA, Bozarth MA (1987). A psychomotor stimulant theory of addiction. *Psychol Rev* 94:469–492.

14. Cazala P (1986). Self-stimulation behavior can be elicited from various 'aversive' brain structures. *Behav Brain Res* 22:163–171.

15. Di Chiara G, Imperato A (1985). Ethanol preferentially stimulates dopamine release in the nucleus accumbens of freely moving rats. *Eur J Pharmacol* 115:131–132.

16. Gessa GL, Muntoni F, Collu M, Vargiu L, Mereu G (1985). Low doses of ethanol activate dopaminergic neurons in the ventral tegmental area. *Brain Res* 348:201–203.

17. Gysling K, Wang RY (1983). Morphine-induced activation of A10 dopamine neurons in the rat. *Brain Res* 277:119–127.

18. Esposito RU, Kornetsky C (1978). Opioids and rewarding brain stimulation. *Neurosci Biobehav Rev* 2:115–122.

19. Hubner CB, Bain GT, Kornetsky C (1987). The combined effects of morphine and d-amphetamine on the threshold for brain stimulation reward. *Pharmacol Biochem Behav* 28:311–315.

20. Morley JE, Levine AS, Yim GK, Lowy MT (1983). Opioid modulation of appetite. *Neurosci Biobehav Rev* 7:281–305.

21. Mucha RF, Iversen SD (1986). Increased food intake after opioid microinjections into nucleus accumbens and ventral tegmental area of rat. *Brain Res* 397:214–224.

22. Jackson HC, Sewell RDE (1985). Are δ-opioid receptors involved in the regulation of food and water intake? *Neuropharmacology* 24:885–888.

23. Cooper SJ (1984). Sweetness, reward and analgesia. *Trends Pharmacol Sci* 5:322–323.

24. Dum J, Gramsch C, Herz A (1983). Activation of hypothalamic β-endorphin pools by reward induced by highly palatable food. *Pharmacol Biochem Behav* 18:443–447.

25. Le Magnen J, Marfaing-Jallat P, Miceli D, Devos M (1980). Pain modulating and reward systems: A single brain mechanism? *Pharmacol Biochem Behav* 12:729–733.

26. Seeger TF, Carlson KR, Nazzaro JM (1981). Pentobarbital induces a naloxone-reversible decrease in mesolimbic self-stimulation threshold. *Pharmacol Biochem Behav* 15:583–586.

27. Wise RA (1980). Action of drugs of abuse on brain reward systems. *Pharmacol Biochem Behav* 13(Suppl 1):213–223.

28. Waszczak BL, Walters JR (1980). Intravenous GABA agonist administration stimulates firing of A10 dopaminergic neurons. *Eur J Pharmacol* 66:141–144.

29. Griffiths RR, Bigelow GE, Liebson IA (1986). Human coffee drinking: Reinforcing and physical dependence producing effects of caffeine. *J Pharmacol Exp Ther* 239:416–425.
30. de Wit H, Uhlenhuth EH, Johanson CE (1986). Individual differences in the reinforcing and subjective effects of amphetamine and diazepam. *Drug Alc Depend* 16:341–360.
31. Swerdlow NR, Koob GF (1984). Restrained rats learn amphetamine-conditioned locomotion, but not place preference. *Psychopharmacology* 84:163–166.
32. Carr GD, Phillips AG, Fibiger HC (1988). Independence of amphetamine reward from locomotor stimulation demonstrated by conditioned place preference. *Psychopharmacology* 94:221–226.
33. Rossi NA, Reid LD (1976). Affective states associated with morphine injections. *Physiol Psychol* 4:269–274.
34. Mucha RF, van der Kooy D, O'Shaughnessy M, Bucenieks P (1982). Drug reinforcement studied by the use of place conditioning in rat. *Brain Res* 243:91–105.
35. Stewart RB, Grupp LA (1985). Some determinants of the motivational properties of ethanol in the rat: Concurrent administration of food or social stimuli. *Psychopharmacology* 87:43–50.
36. van der Kooy D, Mucha RF, O'Shaughnessy M, Bucenieks P (1982). Reinforcing effects of brain microinjections of morphine revealed by conditioned place preference. *Brain Res* 243:107–117.
37. Mucha RF, Herz A (1986). Preference conditioning produced by opioid active and inactive isomers of levorphanol and morphine in rat. *Life Sci* 38:241–249.
38. Mucha RF, Millan MJ, Herz A (1985). Aversive properties of naloxone in non-dependent (naive) rats may involve blockade of central β-endorphin. *Psychopharmacology* 86:281–285.
39. Mucha RF, Walker MJK (1987). Aversive property of opioid receptor blockade in drug-naive mice. *Psychopharmacology* 93:483–488.
40. Amalric M, Cline EJ, Martinez JL Jr, Bloom FE, Koob GF (1987). Rewarding properties of β-endorphin as measured by conditioned place preference. *Psychopharmacology* 91:14–19.
41. Bardo MT, Neisewander JL (1987). Chronic naltrexone supersensitizes the reinforcing and locomotor activating effects of morphine. *Pharmacol Biochem Behav* 28:267–273.
42. Mucha RF, Herz A (1985). Motivational properties of kappa and mu opioid receptor agonists studied with place and taste preference conditioning. *Psychopharmacology* 86:274–280.
43. Spyraki C, Fibiger HC (1988). A role for the mesolimbic dopamine system in the reinforcing properties of diazepam. *Psychopharmacology* 94:133–137.
44. De Witte P, Bada MF (1983). Self-stimulation and alcohol administered orally or intraperitoneally. *Exp Neurol* 82:675–682.
45. Schaefer GJ, Richardson WR, Bonsall RW, Michael RP (1988). Brain self-stimulation, locomotor activity and tissue concentrations of ethanol in male rats. *Drug Alc Depend* 21:67–75.
46. Morse WH, Kelleher RT (1977). Determinants of reinforcement and punishment. In WK Honig, JER Staddon, eds. *Handbook of Operant Behavior,* 2nd ed. Appleton, New York, pp 174–200.

47. Gallistel CR (1986). The role of the dopaminergic projections in MFB self-stimulation. *Behav Brain Res* 22:97–105.
48. Ljungberg T (1987). Blockade by neuroleptics of water intake and operant responding for water in the rat: Anhedonia, motor deficit, or both? *Pharmacol Biochem Behav* 27:341–350.
49. Cunningham CL (1981). Spatial aversion conditioning with ethanol. *Pharmacol Biochem Behav* 14:263–264.
50. Stewart RB, Grupp LA (1981). An investigation of the interaction between the reinforcing properties of food and ethanol using the place preference paadigm. *Progr Neuropsychopharmacol* 5:609–613.
51. van der Kooy D, O'Shaughnessy M, Mucha RF, Kalant H (1983). Motivational properties of ethanol in naive rats as studied by place conditioning. *Pharmacol Biochem Behav* 19:441–445.
52. Mucha RF, Iversen SD (1984). Reinforcing properties of morphine and naloxone revealed by conditioned place preferences. *Psychopharmacology* 82:241–247.
53. File SE (1986). Aversive and appetitive properties of anxiogenic and anxiolytic agents. *Behav Brain Res* 21:189–194.
54. Ator NA, Griffiths RR (1987). Self-administration of barbiturates and benzodiazepines: A review. *Pharmacol Biochem Behav* 27:391–398.
55. Grupp LA, Stewart RB (1983). Active and passive avoidance behaviour in rats produced by IV infusions of ethanol. *Psychopharmacology* 79:318–321.
56. Stewart RB, Grupp LA (1986). Conditioned place aversion mediated by orally self-administered ethanol. *Pharmacol Biochem Behav* 24:1369–1375.
57. Beardsley PM, Meisch RA (1981). A precision drinking device for rats tested with water, etonitazene, and ethanol. *Pharmacol Biochem Behav* 14:871–876.
58. Grant KA, Samson HH (1986). The induction of oral ethanol self-administration by contingent ethanol delivery. *Drug Alc Depend* 16:361–368.
59. Stiglick A, Woodworth I (1984). Increase in ethanol consumption in rats due to caloric deficit. *Alcohol* 1:413–415.
60. Carroll ME (1985). The role of food deprivation in the maintenance and reinstatement of cocaine-seeking behavior in rats. *Drug Alc Depend* 16:95–109.
61. Goeders NE, Smith JE (1983). Cortical dopaminergic involvement in cocaine reinforcement. *Science* 221:773–775.
62. Goeders NE, Dworkin SI, Smith JE (1986). Neuropharmacological assessment of cocaine self-administration into the medial prefrontal cortex. *Pharmacol Biochem Behav* 24:1429–1440.
63. Woolverton WL (1986). Effects of a D_1 and a D_2 dopamine antagonist on the self-administration of cocaine and piribedil by rhesus monkeys. *Pharmacol Biochem Behav* 24:531–535.
64. Corrigall WA (1987). Heroin self-administration: Effects of antagonist treatment in lateral hypothalamus. *Pharmacol Biochem Behav* 27:693–700.
65. Corrigall WA, Vaccarino FJ (1988). Antagonist treatment in nucleus accumbens or periaqueductal grey affects heroin self-administration. *Pharmacol Biochem Behav* 30:443–450.
66. Ettenberg A, Pettit HO, Bloom FE, Koob GF (1982). Heroin and cocaine intravenous self-administration in rats: Mediation by separate neural systems. *Psychopharmacology* 78:204–209.

67. Pettit HO, Ettenberg A, Bloom FE, Koob GF (1984). Destruction of dopamine in the nucleus accumbens selectively attenuates cocaine but not heroin self-administration in rats. *Psychopharmacology* 84:167–173.

68. Mackey WB, van der Kooy D (1985). Neuroleptics block the positive reinforcing effects of amphetamine but not of morphine as measured by place conditioning. *Pharmacol Biochem Behav* 22:101–106.

69. Kalivas PW, Bronson M (1985). Mesolimbic dopamine lesions produce an augmented behavioral response to enkephalin. *Neuropharmacology* 24:931–936.

70. Druhan JP, Martin-Iverson MT, Wilkie DM, Fibiger HC, Phillips AG (1987). Dissociation of dopaminergic and non-dopaminergic substrates for cues produced by electrical stimulation of the ventral tegmental area. *Pharmacol Biochem Behav* 28:251–259.

71. Druhan JP, Martin-Iverson MT, Wilkie DM, Fibiger HC, Phillips AG (1987). Differential effects of physostigmine on cues produced by electrical stimulation of the ventral tegmental area using two discrimination procedures. *Pharmacol Biochem Behav* 28:261–265.

72. Smith JE, Lane JD (1983). Brain neurotransmitter turnover correlated with morphine self-administration. In JE Smith, JD Lane, eds. *The Neurobiology of Opiate Reward Processes*, Elsevier, Amsterdam, pp 361–402.

73. Kalant OJ (1973). *The Amphetamines: Toxicity and Addiction.* 2nd ed. University of Toronto Press, Toronto.

74. Jones RT (1984). The pharmacology of cocaine. In J Grabowski, ed. *Cocaine: Pharmacology, Effects, and Treatment of Abuse.* National Institute on Drug Abuse, Washington DC, pp 34–53.

75. Kalant OJ (1987). *Maier's Cocaine Addiction (Der Kokainismus).* Addiction Research Foundation, Toronto.

76. Huston JP, Tomaz C (1986). Subtelencephalic locale of reinforcement and learning: Looking for the minimal necessary structures. *Behav Brain Res* 22:153–161.

77. Murray RM, Clifford CA, Gurling, HMD (1983). Twin and adoption studies. How good is the evidence for a genetic role? In M Galanter, ed. Recent Developments in Alcoholism, vol 1. Plenum, New York, pp 25–48.

78. Petersen DR (1983). Pharmacogenetic approaches to the neuropharmacology of ethanol. In M Galanter, ed. *Recent Developments in Alcoholism,* vol 1. Plenum, New York, pp 49–69.

79. Deitrich RA, Spuhler K (1984). Genetics of alcoholism and alcohol actions. In RG Smart, HD Cappell, FB Glaser, Y Israel, H Kalant, RE Popham, W Schmidt, EM Sellers, eds. *Recent Advances in Alcohol and Drug Problems,* vol. 8. Plenum, New York, pp 47–98.

80. Volicer L, Volicer BJ, D'Angelo N (1985). Assessment of genetic predisposition to alcoholism in male alcoholics. *Alc Alcoholism* 20:63–68.

81. Schuckit MA (1985). Behavioral effects of alcohol in sons of alcoholics. In M Galanter, ed. *Recent Developments in Alcoholism,* vol 3. Plenum, New York, pp 11–19.

82. Pollock VE, Volavka J, Goodwin DW, Mednick SA, Gabrielli, WF, Knop J, Schulsinger F (1983). The EEG after alcohol administration in men at risk for alcoholism. *Arch Gen Psychiatry* 40:857–861.

83. Begleiter H, Porjesz B, Bihari B, Kissin B (1984). Event-related brain potentials in boys at risk for alcoholism. *Science* 225:1493–1496.

84. Eriksson K (1968). Genetic selection for voluntary alcohol consumption in the albino rat. *Science* 159:739–741.
85. Mardones J, Segovia-Riquelme N (1983). Thirty-two years of selection of rats by ethanol preference: UChA and UChB strains. *Neurobehav Toxicol Teratol* 5:171–178.
86. Eriksson K, Rusi M (1981). Finnish selection studies on alcohol-related behaviors: General outline. In GE McClearn, RA Deitrich, VG Erwin, eds. *Development of Animal Models as Pharmacogenetic Tools*. US Department of Health and Human Services, Washington, DC, pp 87–117.
87. Li T-K, Lumeng L, McBride WJ, Murphy JM (1987). Rodent lines selected for factors affecting alcohol consumption. *Alcohol & Alcoholism* Suppl. 1:91–96.
88. Belknap JK (1980). Genetic factors in the effects of alcohol: Neurosensitivity, functional tolerance and physical dependence. In H Rigter, JC Crabbe, eds. *Alcohol Tolerance and Dependence*. Elsevier, New York, pp 157–180.
89. Goldman D, Lister RG, Crabbe JC (1987). Mapping of a putative genetic locus determining ethanol intake in the mouse. *Brain Res* 420:220–226.
90. Dymshitz J, Lieblich I (1987). Opiate reinforcement and naloxone aversion, as revealed by place preference paradigm, in two strains of rats. *Psychopharmacology* 92:473–477.
91. George FR (1987). Genetic and environmental factors in ethanol self-administration. *Pharmacol Biochem Behav* 27:379–384.
92. Crabbe JC, Kosobud A (1986). Sensitivity and tolerance to ethanol in mice bred to be genetically prone or resistant to ethanol withdrawal seizures. *J Pharmacol Exp Ther* 239:327–333.
93. Cloninger CR (1987). Neurogenetic adaptive mechanisms in alcoholism. *Science* 236:410–416.
94. Johanson CE (1975). Pharmacological and environmental variables affecting drug preference in Rhesus monkeys. *Pharmacol Rev* 27:343–355.
95. Kautz M, Jeffreys R, McBride S, Pournaghash S, Schwartz M, Titley T, Wachsman A, Mastropaolo JP, Riley AL (1987). The sensitivity of conditioned taste aversions as a behavioral baseline to assess the discriminative stimulus properties of naloxone. *Neurosci Abstr* 13:1037.
96. Martin GM, Bechara A, van der Kooy D (1987). Dissociation of morphine's discriminative stimulus properties from its motivational properties. *Neurosci Abstr* 13:1546.
97. Mastropaolo JP, Moskowitz KH, Dacanay RJ, Riley AL (1986). Conditioned taste aversions in rats as a behavioral baseline for the assessment of the stimulus properties of phencyclidine. *Neurosci Abstr* 12:912.
98. Revusky S, Coombes S, Pohl RW (1982). Drug states as discriminative stimuli in a flavor aversion learning experiment. *J Comp Physiol Psychol* 96:200–211.
99. Bartoletti M, Gaiardi M, Gubellini C, Bacchi A, Babbini M (1985). Cross-sensitization to the excitatory effect of morphine in post-dependent rats. *Neuropharmacology* 24:889–893.
100. Kalant H, LeBlanc AE, Gibbins RJ (1971). Tolerance to, and dependence on, some non-opiate psychotropic drugs. *Pharmacol Rev* 23:135–191.

101. Krasnegor NA (1978). *Behavioral Tolerance: Research and Treatment Implications*, NIDA Research Monograph 18. US Department of Health and Human Services, Washington, DC.
102. Rigter H, Crabbe JC Jr, eds (1980). *Alcohol Tolerance and Dependence* Elsevier/North-Holland, New York.
103. Sharp CW, ed (1984). *Mechanisms of Tolerance and Dependence*, NIDA Research Monograph 54. US Department of Health and Human Services, Washington, DC.
104. Downs DA, Woods JH, Llewellyn ME (1975). The behavioural pharmacology of addiction: Some conceptual and methodological foci. In HD Cappell, AE LeBlanc, eds. *Biological and Behavioural Approaches to Drug Dependence*. Addiction Research Foundation, Toronto, pp 53–71.
105. McCown TJ, Barrett RJ (1980). Development of tolerance to the rewarding effects of self-administered S(+)-amphetamine. *Pharmacol Biochem Behav* 12:137–141.
106. Barrett RJ (1985). Behavioral approaches to individual differences in substance abuse. Drug-taking behavior. In M Galizio, SA Maisto, eds. *Determinants of Substance Abuse: Biological, Psychological and Environmental Factors*. Plenum, New York, pp 125–175.
107. McQuarrie DG, Fingl E (1958). Effects of single doses and chronic administration of ethanol on experimental seizures in mice. *J Pharmacol Exp Ther* 124:264–271.
108. Hughes PH, Venulet J, U Khant, Medina Mora ME, Navaratnam V, Poshyachinda V, Rootman I, Salan R, Wadud KA (1980). *Core Data for Epidemiological Studies of Non-Medical Drug Use*. World Health Organization, Geneva.
109. Lau, H-H (1975). Cost of alcoholic beverages as a determinant of alcohol consumption. In RJ Gibbins, Y Israel, H Kalant, RE Popham, W Schmidt, RG Smart, eds. *Research Advances in Alcohol and Drug Problems*, vol 2. Wiley-Biomedical, New York, pp 211–245.
110. Bunce R (1976). *Alcoholic Beverage Consumption, Beverage Prices and Income in California 1952–1975*. Report No. 6, June. State Office of Alcoholism, Sacramento, CA.
111. Adrian M, Ferguson BS (1986). The influence of income on the consumption of alcohol in Ontario: A cross-section study. In A Carmi, S Schneider, eds. *Drugs and Alcohol (Medicolegal Library 6)*. Springer-Verlag, New York, pp 151–157.
112. Bruun K, Edwards G, Lumio M, Mäkelä K, Tan L, Popham RE, Room R, Schmidt W, Skog OJ, Sulkunen P, Österberg E (1975). *Alcohol Control Policies in Public Health Perspective*. Finnish Foundation for Alcohol Studies, vol 25. Finnish Foundation, Helsinki.
113. Babor TF, Mendelson JH, Greenberg I, Kuehnle J (1978). Experimental analysis of the "happy hour": Effect of purchase price on alcohol consumption. *Psychopharmacology* 58:35–41.
114. Gold MS, Washton AM, Dackis CA (1985). Cocaine abuse: Neurochemistry, phenomenology, and treatment. In NJ Kozel, EH Adams, eds. *Cocaine Use in America: Epidemiologic and Clinical Perspectives*. NIDA Research Monograph 61. US Department of Health and Human Services, Washington, DC, pp 130–150.

115. Anonymous (1987). 'Precipitous' increase in crack complications. *The Journal* 16(7):5, July. Addiction Research Foundation, Toronto.
116. Novotny TE, Lynn WR, eds (1988). *The Health Consequences of Smoking: Nicotine Addiction, a Report of the Surgeon General.* US Department of Health and Human Services, Washington, DC, pp 181–192.
117. Hatsukami DK, Dahlgren L, Zimmerman R, Hughes JR (1988). Symptoms of tobacco withdrawal from total cigarette cessation versus partial cigarette reduction. *Psychopharmacology* 94:242–247.
118. Griffiths RR, Woodson PP (1988). Reinforcing properties of caffeine: Studies in humans and laboratory animals. *Pharmacol Biochem Behav* 29:419–427.
119. Griffiths RR, Woodson PP (1988). Caffeine physical dependence: A review of human and laboratory animal studies. *Psychopharmacology* 94:437–451.
120. Ferrence RG (1988). *The Diffusion of Cigarette Smoking: An Exploratory Analysis.* Ph.D. dissertation. University of Western Ontario, London, Canada.
121. Skog O-J (1986). The long waves of alcohol consumption: A social network perspective on cultural change. *Soc Networks* 8:1–32.

CHAPTER 2

Neuroanatomical and Neurochemical Substrates of Drug-Seeking Behavior: Overview and Future Directions

Stanley J. Watson, Keith A. Trujillo,
James P. Herman, and Huda Akil

The focus of this volume, *Molecular and Cellular Aspects of the Drug Addictions,* addresses but one perspective of an admittedly complex biological, psychological, and social phenomenon: the administration of drugs for nonmedical reasons. It is readily acknowledged that, in the human, "drug abuse" and "addiction" involve interactions between biological, psychological, and social dimensions. However, it is also readily apparent from both human and animal research that much can be discussed concerning the biological dimension; drugs are self-administered because of their effects on biological systems in the brain. Moreover, research is leading us steadily closer to the specific neuro-chemical, neuroanatomical, molecular, and cellular actions that are important in the self-administration of drugs.

Because of the many social, cultural, and emotional connotations, as well as the use and misuse of the term by the layman, the term "addiction" can mean different things to different people. Addiction oftentimes refers to a condition arrived at through the habitual use of drugs and is therefore most often confused with some of the consequences of chronic administration of drugs, including tolerance and physical dependence. It is therefore important in any discussion of the subject either to use an alternate term or to provide a careful operational definition for the term "addiction." Because of the potential confusion with tolerance and dependence, we prefer not to use "addiction" in the present discussion. Other descriptors such as "recreational use of drugs" or "nonmedical use of drugs" either sound trivial or are unwieldly for general use. Still other terms, such as "drug abuse" or related descriptors, are emotion-laden and are therefore difficult to use in an objective discussion. In fact, the World Health Organization has suggested that the term "abuse" no longer be use in reference to drugs on the grounds that it represents a value judgment rather than an operational definition (1). Probably the easiest way around this problem is to simply refer to the drugs in question as "self-administered" drugs. This terminology not only describes the fact that these drugs are considered to be "addictive" because they are self-administered by humans for reasons other than their medical value, but also fits well with studies in behavioral pharmacology that examine the self-administration of drugs in animals.

The purpose of this chapter is to explore the neurochemical and neuroanatomical systems involved in the self-administration of drugs. Our primary focus is on examining the self-administration of opioid compounds. However, it is very difficult to enter a complete discussion of opioid self-administration without discussing other self-administered drugs—most notably, the psychomotor stimulants. Therefore, although the weight of the chapter will examine opioids, we will also spend some time examining psychomotor stimulant self-administration. We will begin by briefly discussing the two major theoretic perspectives that researchers use in the study of this behavior: positive reinforcement and negative reinforcement. We will then review studies relevant to the positive reinforcing aspects of both psychomotor stimulants and opioids, including behavioral, pharmacological, neurochemical, and, in considerable detail, neuroanatomical studies. As discussed below, through our review of this data we have come to recognize a "limbic-motor reinforcement circuit" that we believe may be important not only in the self-administration of drugs but also in brain mechanisms of positive reinforcement. Following our discussion of the positive reinforcing aspects of self-administration, we will overview recent research pertinent to the negative reinforcing actions of self-administered drugs. Finally, with this background, we will present our perspectives on the neural systems that appear to be involved in drug self-administration and propose future studies that we believe may help provide knowledge needed to understand and treat self-administration of psychoactive drugs more effectively.

Theoretical Perspective: Positive Versus Negative Reinforcement

The concepts of operant psychology (2) have played an important role in the theoretical approach to studies of drug self-administration. According to operant psychology, behavior is controlled by its consequences. A consequence that leads to an increase in behavior, whether it is a positive stimulus or a negative stimulus, is referred to as a reinforcer. A positive reinforcer is a stimulus that can be obtained by a behavioral action and thereby leads to an increase in that behavior. Positive reinforcers are typically associated with positive affective tone, such as euphoria, and are therefore sometimes referred to as rewards. A typical example is a rat lever-pressing for a food pellet; since the rat will repeatedly press the lever in order to obtain the food pellet, the pellet is a positive reinforcer. A negative reinforcer is a stimulus that can be prevented by a behavioral action, and consequently leads to an increase in that behavior. Negative reinforcers are usually associated with negative affective tone. A good example of this is a rat lever-pressing to avoid an electric shock; since the rat will repeatedly lever-press in order to avoid the electric shock, the shock is a negative reinforcer. Negative reinforcement is often confused with punishment. Although negative reinforcement and punishment are both typically associated with negative affect, there is an important difference: Negative reinforcement leads to an increase in the target behavior, whereas punishment leads to a decrease. In our rat model, if pressing of the lever is followed by an electric shock, a decrease in lever pressing will occur. Since the behavioral consequence in this case is a decrease in lever pressing rather than an increase, the electric shock is a punisher rather than a negative reinforcer. The critical concept here has to do with reinforcement. In both positive reinforcement and negative reinforcement the behavioral consequence is the same, an increase in behavior (lever pressing), whereas the controlling stimulus (food pellet or electric shock) and the emotions it evokes are quite different. It is from the theoretical perspectives of positive reinforcement and negative reinforcement that researchers have approached the self-administration of drugs.

Positive Reinforcement and Self-Administration

There are several identifiable classes of self-administered drugs, including psychomotor stimulants, opioids, sedative hypnotics, nicotine, cannabinoids, arylcyclohexamines, and inhalants (3). Although they are seemingly diverse, these groups of drugs can be identified by their common ability to serve as positive reinforcers in humans and experimental animals; each of the drugs in these groups has the ability to control behavior in a manner similar to natural positive reinforcers such as food and water. For example, an experimental animal will press a lever repeatedly, and a human user will go to great lengths in order to self-administer one of these drugs. Recent theories have therefore focused on positive reinforcement to explain the self-administration of drugs. To state that self-administered drugs are positively reinforcing, however, is merely stating the obvious; their effect on behavior identifies these drugs as positive reinforcers. The power of the statement comes into play when it is recognized that there are specialized brain systems that mediate positive reinforcement and that these systems are responsible for the positive reinforcing effects of drugs.

Olds and Milner in 1954, in demonstrating that animals would electrically self-stimulate the brain, provided the first experimental evidence that positive reinforcement was mediated by specific brain systems (4). Natural reinforcers normally gain access to brain reinforcement circuitry by way of the sensory systems, such as olfaction, taste, and vision. In the self-stimulation experiment the animal is given the opportunity to bypass sensory input and directly stimulate the positive reinforcement circuitry of the brain. Electrical brain stimulation is so potently reinforcing that animals will forgo natural reinforcers such as food, water, and sex in order to self-stimulate (5). The electrical self-stimulation experiment can be viewed as a chemical self-administration experiment. Electrical activation of neuronal cell bodies or axons at the tip of the electrode causes release of neurotransmitters from the nerve terminals; it is these substances that are responsible for the reinforcement message. A major focus of research on brain mechanisms of positive reinforcement has therefore been to identify the neurotransmitters that mediate this phenomenon. Evidence suggests that two classes of neurotransmitter—the endogenous opioids and catecholamines—may be primary mediators of positive reinforcement in the brain (6). Significantly, as discussed below, some of the most highly self-administered drugs are known to act by mimicking endogenous opioids (morphine, heroin) or catecholamines (amphetamine, cocaine). It therefore appears that the positive reinforcing actions of self-administered drugs result from their ability to bypass sensory systems and directly access the positive reinforcement circuitry of the brain. In light of the selectivity of neurotransmitters responsible for positive reinforcement, it is not surprising that of the literally millions of natural and synthetic compounds known to humankind, very few are self-administered.

Almost certainly related to the positive reinforcing actions of self-adminsitered drugs are the euphorigenic (pleasure-producing) properties of these compounds. Users have long reported that these drugs produce a pleasurable subjective experience (7). Although recent studies have attempted to quantify the euphorigenic properties of self-administered drugs in humans (8), is it unfortunately impossible to study such a subjective response in the experimental animal. The study of these drugs in animals is therefore left to objective measures of positive reinforcement. Three experimental paradigms important in this field of study are self-administration, conditioned preference, and self-stimulation (Figure 2.1); see Bozarth (8) for excellent reviews of methods. In the self-administration study, the experimental animal (or human subject) performs a nominal task to obtain an injection of drug. In the conditioned preference experiment, a drug is repeatedly paired with a particular environmental cue; when tested later, the approach or avoidance of the animal for that cue determines whether the drug was reinforcing, neutral, or aversive. In the self-stimulation experiment an animal with an electrode implanted in the brain performs a nominal task to stimulate a particular brain site electrically. Although the study of self-stimulation is more fundamentally concerned with brain reinforcement circuitry, this paradigm can also be used to study self-administered drugs; research on self-stimulation has demonstrated that self-administered drugs will spe-

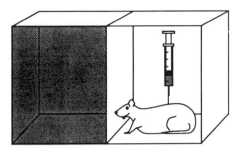

CONDITIONED PLACE PREFERENCE

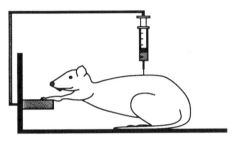

SELF-ADMINISTRATION

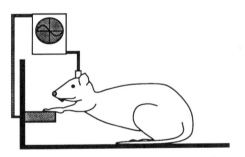

INTRACRANIAL SELF-STIMULATION

FIGURE 2.1. Schematic drawings illustrating the three major experimental paradigms used to study the positive reinforcing actions of self-administered drugs. See text for descriptions.

cifically facilitate self-stimulation behavior. Using these paradigms one can study the positive reinforcing actions of systemic injections of a drug or obtain a reasonable degree of neuroanatomical specificity by injecting the drug directly into a specific brain region. In addition, one can study the effects of various behavioral manipulations, pharmacological manipulations, brain lesions, and so forth, on self-administration, conditioned preference or self-stimulation in order to examine behavioral, neuro-chemical, and neuroanatomical factors involved in the positive rein-forcing actions of a particular drug.

Negative Reinforcement and Self-Administration

Whereas recent theories on the self-administration of drugs have focused on their positive reinforcing actions, earlier theories were built around the concept of negative reinforcement (9–11). These theories focused on tolerance and dependence and, in particular, on the negative reinforcing properties of the withdrawal syndrome. Tolerance refers to a shift in the dose-response curve following treatment with a drug, whereby a higher dose of the drug is needed to obtain a particular effect. Dependence refers to a state following chronic exposure to a drug wherein continued administration of the drug is necessary for "normal" function. If a drug is withdrawn from a dependent subject, a characteristic withdrawal or abstinence syndrome results. According to negative reinforcement theo-ries, drugs are self-administered in order to avoid the aversive conse-quences of the withdrawal syndrome. Several lines of evidence, however, have prompted researchers to question the role of negative reinforcement in drug self-administration. For example, self-administration of drugs can occur in the absence of tolerance or physical dependence in both animals (12–15) and humans (16,17). In contrast, tolerance and physical depen-dence can be observed following exposure to drugs, such as propranalol or nitrates, that are not readily self-administered (18). Thus, although tolerance and dependence often occur after repeated administration of self-administered drugs, these properties are not predictive of, or neces-sary for, self-administration.

It should be noted, however, that dependence can be an important factor in the maintenance of self-administration. The aversiveness of the abstinence syndrome can indeed serve as a powerful negative reinforcer for continued self-administration of drug after the subject has become dependent. In this respect it is important to distinguish between the initiation and the maintenance of self-administration. Although the initia-tion depends primarily on the positive reinforcing properties of a drug, the maintenance of self-administration in a dependent subject depends on both positive and negative reinforcement (19–21). The importance of negative reinforcement becomes readily apparent in accounts from opioid addicts and clinicians who treat these patients. These accounts often refer to the powerfully aversive emotions experienced during withdrawal, including profound anxiety and a "craving" for more drug. The aversive emotions triggered by the withdrawal syndrome apparently contribute more to negative reinforcement than the physical symptoms. The physical symptoms have been referred to as no worse than a bad case of the flu (22). However, the anxiety and craving that accompany the physical symptoms appear to be powerfully motivating forces for continued self-administration. It is therefore incumbent on researchers to learn more about the negative reinforcing aspects of the withdrawal syndrome in order to provide a fuller understanding of self-administration of drugs.

As noted above, it is impossible to study subjective emotional responses in an experimental animal. The study of the withdrawal syndrome has therefore been left to objective measures. One method used by researcher has been to use chronic injections of a self-administered drug and then to quantify the physical symptoms following withdrawal of that drug or following administration of an antagonist (23,24). Conversely, one can administer agonist drugs during abstinence to examine whether the agonist will suppress any of the physical symptoms of withdrawal. Some degree of neuroanatomical specificity can be achieved using either of these paradigms by microinjecting the agonist or antagonist directly into specific brain sites. It should be noted, however, that the physical symptoms of withdrawal are probably not the best assessment of the aversiveness of the withdrawal syndrome. These symptoms may simply be side effects of drug withdrawal that have little to do with the powerfully aversive experience. It is therefore better to measure more direct signs of aversion, such as escape responses (23,24) or conditioned place aversions (25) during withdrawal.

Positive Reinforcing Actions of Self-Administered Drugs

In the following discussion we will review research on the neural substrates responsible for the positive reinforcing actions of opioids and psychomotor stimulants. Opioid compounds and psychomotor stimulants contain some of the most highly reinforcing compounds known to humankind. Moreover, there are important similarities and even overlaps between the systems involved in the reinforcing actions of these drugs. In fact, as discussed below, some researchers have suggested that the positive reinforcing actions of opioid compounds occur by activating the same systems activated by psychomotor stimulants. Others, however, disagree with this assessment and suggest that the systems, though closely associated, are distinguishable. Following our review of the behavioral pharmacology of psychomotor stimulant and opioid positive reinforcement, we will examine in detail the neuroanatomical sites and circuits that appear to mediate the positive reinforcing actions of these drugs.

Neurochemical Actions of Psychomotor Stimulants

The psychomotor stimulants, including amphetamine, amphetamine-like stimulants, and cocaine, comprise a group of drugs with similar neurochemical and behavioral actions. These drugs have been self-administered by humans throughout recorded history, and their current popularity has made them the subject of intense political and media concern. Since amphetamine and cocaine are the most widely self-administered as well as the most widely studied of these compounds, the present discussion will deal primarily with these two drugs. It should be kept in mind, however, that all the drugs in this class have very similar, if not identical, mechanisms of action.

The fact that the psychomotor stimulants have very important structural similarities with the catecholamines, dopamine, and norepinephrine gives an important clue as to their mechanism of action (Figure 2.2). Amphetamine, for example, stimulates release of dopamine and norepinephrine from nerve terminals, blocks neuronal reuptake of the catecholamines, and inhibits the catecholamine metabolic enzyme monoamine oxidase. Cocaine is a potent inhibitor of neuronal reuptake of the catecholamines; however, unlike amphetamine, it does not actively stimulate the release of dopamine and norepinephrine (26). Although the molecular sites of action for these drugs have not been clearly identified, intriguing evidence suggests that the stimulants may produce their effects on catecholamine neurons by mimicking the actions of the endogenous compound β-phenylethylamine (27).

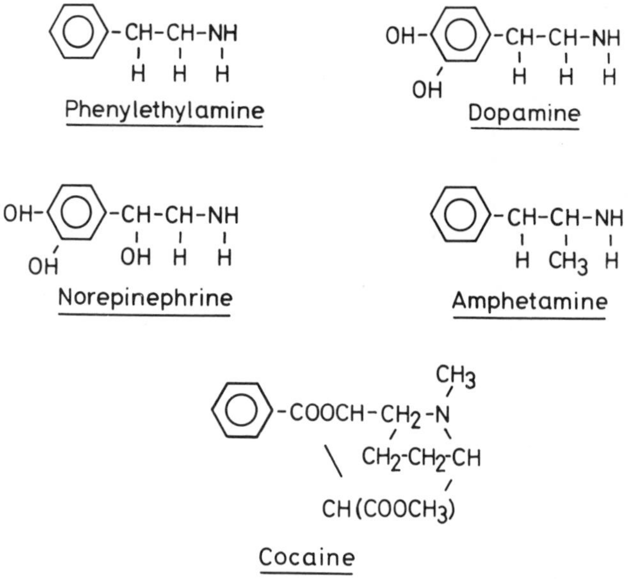

FIGURE 2.2. Chemical structures for phenylethylamine, dopamine, norepinephrine, amphetamine, and cocaine. Note the striking structural similarities between the endogenous neurotransmitters dopamine and norepinephrine and the psychomotor stimulants amphetamine and cocaine.

Reinforcing Actions of Psychomotor Stimulants

The potent actions of psychomotor stimulants on catecholamine neurons suggests that dopamine and/or norepinephrine might mediate the reinforcing actions of these drugs. The bulk of the literature examining catecholamines and reinforcement indicates that release of dopamine, rather than norepinephrine, is primarily responsible for psychomotor stimulant reinforcement (28,29). This hypothesis is supported by the fact that dopamine receptor antagonists but not noradrenergic antagonists will disrupt systemic self-administration of stimulant drugs (30–34), as well as conditioned place preferences produced by these compounds (35–38). In addition, studies on human subjects suggest that amphetamine-dependent euphoria is attenuated by dopamine receptor blockade, but not blockade of noradrenergic receptors (39). Studies using selective lesions of catecholamine neurons support a role for dopamine in psychomotor stimulant reinforcement, and help to identify the nucleus accumbens (NACC) as an important site of action; lesions of this nucleus with 6-hydroxydopamine disrupt the reinforcing actions of both amphetamine and cocaine (35,40–42). Experiments in which these drugs are injected directly into specific brain regions of rats also suggest a role for NACC dopamine in the reinforcing actions of amphetamine (43–47) (see Figure 2.3); however, conflicting results are obtained for cocaine. Although some studies suggest that cocaine is reinforcing when injected into the NACC (48), others dispute these results and suggest that medial prefrontal cortex (MPC) is responsible for the reinforcing actions of this drug (49–51) (Figure 2.3). Interestingly, rats will self-administer dopamine directly into either the NACC (52) or the MPC (50,51). More specific pharmacological studies suggest that, at least in the case of cocaine, the reinforcing message may be mediated by the D2, rather than the D1 dopamine receptor (50,51,53; see also 54). However, recent studies demonstrating that D1 receptor activation is necessary for the expression of D2 receptor effects (55) suggests that activation of both receptor types may be involved in reinforcement.

In summary, it appears that release of dopamine in the NACC is responsible for the reinforcing actions of amphetamine and amphetamine-like stimulants. While dopamine release is also responsible for the reinforcing actions of cocaine, it is currently unclear as to whether the MPC or the NACC (or both) is the primary site of action. It will be considerable interest to clarify whether amphetamine and cocaine produce reinforcement by acting at the same or distinct brain loci. Despite their possible similarities or differences, however, it appears that the release of dopamine in forebrain regions is the critical neurochemical mechanism responsible for the self-administration of these drugs (see Figure 2.3). Interestingly, studies demonstrate that the NACC is also the primary site of action for the locomotor activating effects of psychomotor stimulants (56,57). The association between locomotor activation and

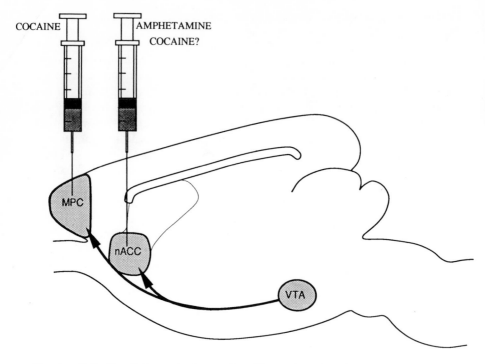

FIGURE 2.3. Saggital rat brain section illustrating the brain sites at which psychomotor stimulants are positively reinforcing. Research is fairly clear in demonstrating a critical role for dopamine nerve terminals in the nucleus accumbens (nACC) in the positive reinforcing actions of amphetamine. There is controversy as to whether the nACC or the medial prefrontal cortex (MPC) (or perhaps both) mediate the reinforcing actions of cocaine. Arrows depict the mesocorticolimbic dopamine pathway projecting from the ventral tegmental area (VTA) to the nACC and the MPC.

reinforcement may offer a potentially valuable tool with which to attempt to understand self-administered drugs and will therefore be discussed in more detail below.

A note of caution is in order, lest we become overly confident in our understanding of the systems underlying the reinforcing actions of psychomotor stimulants. Several studies suggest that the reinforcing actions of amphetamine (58–61) and cocaine (62,63) can be disrupted by administration of the opioid receptor antagonist naloxone. In addition, we have recently obtained evidence that acute injections of amphetamine cause depletion of dynorphins in rat forebrain regions, suggesting that amphetamine causes release of these endogenous opioids (Trujillo, Day, and Akil, in preparation). Such evidence raises the possibility that release of dynorphin may, in some situations, mediate the reinforcing actions of psychomotor stimulants. Furthermore, although dopamine appears to play an important, perhaps even critical, role in psychomotor stimulant reinforcement, one cannot completely dismiss a possible role for norepinephrine. Recent research suggests that noradrenergic agonists, including norepinephrine itself, are reinforcing (64–66). These findings suggest that the systems we are dealing with may be more complex than is sometimes acknowledged. Hence researchers should be open to new, sometimes paradoxical results.

Neurochemical Aspects of Opioids

Opioid compounds, like psychomotor stimulants, have been used by humans throughout recorded history for both medicinal and non-medicinal purposes. Despite this long history of use, the neurochemical systems responsible for the actions of these drugs have been elucidated only in the past 15 years. Exogenously administered opioid drugs produce their physiological effects by activating opioid receptors, mimicking the actions of endogenous opioid peptides. As is currently recognized, the endogenous opioid systems are comprised by at least three different receptor types and numerous neuroactive peptides. To fully appreciate the role of these systems in self-administration behavior, it is important to understand their complexities and subtleties. Therefore, before examining the reinforcing actions of opioid compounds, we will review what is currently known about endogenous opioid peptides and receptors.

There are currently three recognized endogenous opioid peptide families—the proenkephalin family (PROENK), the proopiomelanocortin family (POMC), and the prodynorphin family (PRODYN), each the product of a distinct gene and precursor peptide (Figure 2.4). Each of the peptides in these families contain the amino terminal, five amino acid "opioid core" consisting of either Tyr-Tyr-Gly-Gly-Phe-Met (met-enkephalin) or Tyr-Gly-Gly-Phe-Leu (leu-enkephalin), with unique carboxy terminal extensions. The peptides are liberated from their respective precursors by trypsin-like cleavage at double basic amino acid residues (lysine-arginine or lysine-lysine).

Met-enkephalin and leu-enkephalin were the first opioid peptides isolated and characterized, identified by their ability to mimic the actions of morphine in *in vitro* tissue assays (67). These peptides consist of the five amino acid opioid core without carboxy terminal extensions (see above). The enkephalins are products of the PROENK precursor, which contains within it four copies of met-enkephalin, two copies of met-enkephalin extended at the carboxy terminus, and one copy of leu-enkephalin (68,69). This precursor can thus generate met-enkephalin, met-enkephalin-Arg^6-Phe^7, met-enkephalin-Arg^6-Gly^7-Leu^8, and leu-enkephalin. In addition, some of these sequences may appear linked together in endogenously generated peptides: peptide F contains two

40   S.J. Watson, et al

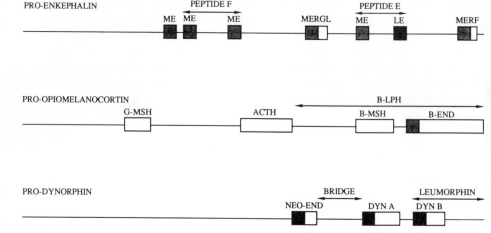

FIGURE 2.4. Schematic representation of the three opioid precursors and their peptide products. Shaded regions represent the met-enkephalin sequence, while black regions represent the leu-enkephalin sequence. ACTH = adrenocorticotropin; B-END = β-endorphin; B-LPH = β-lipotropin; B-MSH = β-melanocyte stimulating hormone; BRIDGE = bridge peptide; DYN A = dynorphin A; DYN B = dynorphin B; G-MSH = γ- melanocyte-stimulating hormone; LE = leu-enkephalin; ME = met-enkephalin; MERF = met-enkephalin-arginine[6]-phenylalanine[7]; MERGL= met-enkephalin-arginine[6]-glycine[7]-leucine[8]; LE = leu-enkephalin.

met-enkephalins separated by several intervening amino acids, whereas peptide E contains one met-enkephalin and one leu-enkephalin separated by intervening amino acids (70).

At the time of the discovery of the enkephalins it was noticed that the pituitary peptide β-lipotropin (β-LPH) contained within it the five amino acid sequence for met-enkephalin (67). This led to a closer examination of β-LPH, with the consequent identification of the opioid peptide β-endorphin (71). This 31 amino acid peptide, which contains the met-enkephalin sequence at its amino terminus, is a product of the POMC precursor (72). It is important to note, however, that β-endorphin is not further processed into met-enkephalin. The carboxy terminal amino acids of β-endorphin 1-31 are sometimes cleaved to produce the smaller peptides β-endorphin 1-27 and 1-26, but there is no cleavage signal within this peptide for the production of met-enkephalin. In addition to β-endorphin, as the name pro-opio-melano-cortin suggests, this precursor codes for the nonopioid peptides α-, β-, and γ-*melano*cyte stimulating hormone (MSH) and adreno*cortico*tropin (ACTH).

Avram Goldstein and co-workers, in 1979, isolated a very potent opioid peptide from porcine pituitary, which they called dynorphin (73). This peptide is now known to be a product of the PRODYN precursor (74). This precursor contains within it three domains for production of opioid peptides, each containing the five amino acid sequence for leu-enkephalin at the amino terminus: the dynorphin A domain, the dynorphin B domain, and the neoendorphin domain. Dynorphin A can be processed to a 1-17 or a 1-8 form. Dynorphin B can appear as a 13 amino acid sequence, or a longer 29 amino acid sequence known as leumorphin. Neoendorphin is found either as a 10 amino acid sequence known as α-neoendorphin or a 9 amino acid sequence known as β-neoendorphin. There is currently debate over whether any of the PRODYN-derived peptides might be further processed to the pentapeptide leu-enkephalin. In addition to the opioid peptides, it appears that the PRODYN precursor produces a 23 amino acid nonopioid peptide sometimes referred to as a bridge peptide (75).

Recent evidence suggests that additional endogenous opioids may exist beyond the three recognized opioid peptide families. For example, the isolation of a distinct clone from frog for the opioid peptide dermorphin (76) suggests that a fourth opioid peptide family may exist. In addition, two groups have independently obtained evidence for the presence of morphine and codeine in mammalian tissue, with suggestions that these alkaloids may be produced endogenously (77–79). It is currently too early to comment on the possible physiological significance of these putative endogenous compounds.

In addition to the multiplicity of endogenous opioid compounds, there are multiple receptor sites at which these compounds and exogenous opioids act in order to produce their physiological effects. There are currently three commonly recognized opioid receptor types, each identified by a unique pharmacological profile and anatomical distribution: μ opioid receptors, which are selectively activated by the opioid alkaloid morphine; δ opioid receptors, by met- and leu-enkephalin; and κ opioid receptors, by benzomorphan opioids and dynorphin peptides (80,81). Although not yet widely recognized, evidence suggests that further opioid receptor types may exist (82). Although all three receptor types are generally thought to cause an inhibitory neuronal response, they appear to be differentially coupled to second-messenger systems. Interestingly, the intraneuronal effects of μ- and δ-receptor activation appear to be identical: an increase in potassium conductance, resulting in hyperpolarization, decreased calcium flux, and an inhibition of action potential discharge (83–86). On the other hand, κ-receptor appear to be coupled to calcium channels; activation of these receptors causes a decrease in calcium conductance and inhibition of action potential discharge (87–90). Although a considerable amount of evidence suggests that opioid receptors may be negatively linked to adenylate cyclase in clonal cells lines, the role of adenylate cyclase as a second-messenger system for opioid receptors in brain is not yet clear (91,92).

It should be kept in mind that the μ-, δ-, and κ-receptors do not correspond in a one-to-one relationship, either pharmacologically or anatomically, with the three opioid peptide families. Although there appears to be pharmacological selectively of certain endogenous opioid peptides and exogenous drugs for certain receptors, there is also considerable cross-reactivity; most compounds will recognize all three receptor types in a descending order of affinity. Divergence of receptor activation is thus seen whereby a given peptide can access multiple receptors (see Table 2.1). In contrast, convergence is also exhibited, in the fact that several peptides, even those from different families, can activate a chosen opioid receptor type (see Table 2.1). The actions of a particular compound at a particular brain site will therefore depend on the specific receptor milieu at that site. For example, while dynorphin A 1-17 preferentially activates κ-receptors, it also has the ability to activate μ- or δ-receptors. The actions of this compound will therefore depend on the ratio of κ-, μ-, and δ-receptors at the brain site under investigation.

A further level of complexity in the interactions between opioid peptides and receptors must be considered when studying these systems. Research on the peptide precursors and their potential products reveals that there is considerable flexibility in the posttranslational processing of these precursors. First, different tissues can process the precursors in different ways. For example, POMC cells in the anterior pituitary produce more of the high molecular weight β-LPH than they do β-endorphin (93), while POMC neurons in the brain produce considerably more β-endorphin sized material (94,95). Similarly, whereas anterior pituitary PRODYN cells produce primarily high-molecular-weight intermediates with very small amounts of end products (Day and Akil, in preparation), PRODYN neurons in the brain produce the smaller-sized dynorphin end products, with considerably more dynorphin A 1-8 than 1-17 (96). An additional level of complexity is added by the fact that environmental influences can modify the products resulting from a

TABLE 2.1. Receptor selectivity profiles[a]

Precursor	Peptide	μ	δ	κ
Pro-Enkephalin	Leu-Enk	19	**1.2**	8210
	Met-Enk	9.5	**0.9**	4440
	Met-Enk-Arg^6-Phe^7	**27**	30	145
	Met-Enk-Arg^6-Gly^7-Leu^8	6.4	**4.8**	89
POMC	β-Endorphin	**2.0**	2.7	57
Pro-Dynorphin	Dyn A (1-8)	3.8	5.0	**1.3**
	Dyn A (1-17)	0.7	2.4	**0.12**
	Dyn B	0.7	3.2	**0.12**
	α-Neo-Endorphin	1.3	0.57	**0.20**

[a]For peptides derived from the three opioid precursors. K_i (nM) values from Leslie (211) and Corbett et al (212), are for binding to guinea pig brain membranes. The values in boldface identify the receptors for which each peptide has highest affinity.

particular precursor. Repeated stress changes not only the processing of anterior pituitary POMC but also the ratios of POMC products released from these neurons upon challenge (93). This change in released products suggests that the chronically stressed rat will receive a different receptor activation profile than the unstressed rat when challenged. With respect to dynorphins, repeated injections of amphetamine increase the levels of PRODYN peptide products in the striatum and substantia nigra; however, the relative increase in the 1-17 form is greater than that of 1-8, resulting in an altered dynorphin 1-8 : 1-17 ratio (97). In light of the different receptor affinities for these peptides, it appears that striatal dynorphin neurons in the amphetamine-treated animal may display a different pattern of receptor stimulation than those in the saline-treated animal. Thus different tissues can yield different peptide products by processing the precursors in different ways; in addition, the pattern of products generated by a particular tissue, and the consequent receptor effects, can be altered by experimental manipulations, including injections of self-administered drugs.

Reinforcing Actions of Opioids

That the positive reinforcing effects of opioids are mediated by actions at opioid receptors is demonstrated by studies using the opioid receptor antagonists naloxone and naltrexone. Weeks and Collins reported in 1976 that injections of naloxone would disrupt morphine self-administration in rats (98). This finding is supported by more recent self-administration studies as well as conditioned preference studies (99–104). Not surprisingly, evidence demonstrates that the reinforcing actions of opioids are mediated by brain rather than peripheral opioid receptors (101).

The multiplicity of opioid receptors and their distinct neuroanatomical distributions raise questions as to which receptors and which brain sites are most important for the positive reinforcing actions of opioid compounds. Recent research has begun to answer these questions, with a major focus on the mesolimbic system. However, although research has focused on the mesolimbic system, there is considerable debate in the literature over the specific brain sites and substrates within this system responsible for opioid reinforcement. Some investigators suggest that opioid reinforcement is dependent on activation of mesolimbic dopamine neurons (102,105–107), whereas others suggest that this phenomenon can occur independent of dopaminergic activation (36,42,99,108).

Demonstrations that opioid reinforcement could be attenuated by dopamine receptor blockade (102,105,109) or by lesions of the mesolimbic dopamine pathway (105,106) have led some investigators to suggest that activation of ventral tegmental area (VTA) dopamine neurons is primarily responsible for the positive reinforcing actions of opioid compounds. This hypothesis is supported by both behavioral and physiological evidence demonstrating that opioids can activate midbrain dopamine neurons (110–114). Indeed, opioids are found to be reinforcing when administered directly into the region of VTA dopamine neurons (103,104,115). Considering that release of dopamine in the terminal regions of the meso-limbic pathway is highly reinforcing (see above), it is not surprising that opioid activation of the VTA dopamine neurons is also reinforcing.

Several studies, however, contradict the claim that opioid reinforcement is dependent on a dopaminergic link. In a key experiment, Ettenberg and co-workers found disruption intravenous cocaine self-administration but not heroin self-administration following treatment with dopamine receptor blockers (99), a finding consistent with data from conditioned preference experiments (36). Similarly, disruption of cocaine self-administration but not heroin self-administration was observed following lesions of dopamine nerve terminals in the NACC (42). These findings should not be disturbing, however, since other brain sites appear to be important for opioid positive reinforcement. In addition to the VTA (115), animals have been reported to self-administer opioids directly into the lateral hypothalamus (LH) (116,117) or the NACC (118,119). Results of conditioned preference experiments are consistent with the suggestion that each of these brain regions is important in opioid reinforcement (103,104,120). It therefore appears that multiple sites can mediate the positive reinforcing actions of opioid compounds (see Figure 2.5). Although the conflicting results obtained in studies examining dopaminergic blockade of opioid reinforcement create some confusion, it is possible that subtle methodological differences contribute to the differing results. Perhaps differences in methodology can affect the specific opioid reinforcement site accessed by systemic injections of opioids; whereas some methods may favor the dopamine-dependent VTA, others may favor dopamine-independent sites.

Until recently, agonists and antagonists selective for different opioid receptors have been unavailable. For this reason relatively little progress has been made toward identifying the specific opioid receptor or receptors responsible for the reinforcing actions of opioid compounds. Recent studies, however, have begun to obtain results pertinent to this question. Studies using agonists selective for κ opioid receptors suggest that activation of these receptors is aversive to both laboratory animals (121,122) and human subjects (123). This result is not surprising in light of the dysphoric effects produced by benzomorphan opioids in humans. The aversive consequences of κ-receptor activation suggests that this receptor may be involved in brain mechanisms of negative reinforcement. In contrast, selective activation of μ-receptors (121,122,124) or δ-receptors (124,125) appears to be positively reinforcing. Thus, whereas κ-receptors may be involved in negative reinforcement and aversion, μ and δ opioid

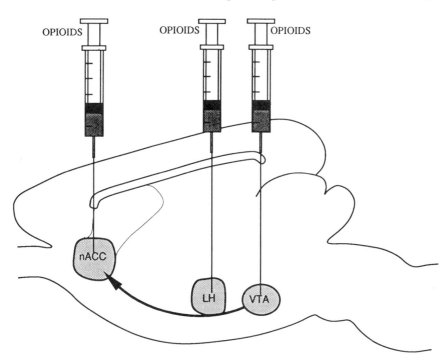

FIGURE 2.5. Saggital rat brain section illustrating the brain sites at which opioids are positively reinforcing. Arrow depicts the mesolimbic dopamine pathway projecting from the ventral tegmental area (VTA) to the nucleus accumbens (nACC). Opioid reinforcement at the level of the VTA appears to result from stimulation of dopamine neurons in this nucleus, with consequent release of dopamine in the nACC. Opioid reinforcement in the nACC may be independent of dopamine. LH = lateral hypothalamus.

receptors may be the molecular sites at which opioids act to produce positive reinforcement. This suggestion is particularly interesting in light of the fact that the intraneuronal coupling of μ- and δ-receptors to second messengers is very similar (see above).

In summary, it would appear that there are multiple mechanisms by which opioids produce their positive reinforcing effects. As in the case of amphetamine-like stimulants, the NACC appears to be an important site of opioid reinforcement. In addition, however, the VTA and the LH are also involved. In the VTA opioid reinforcement results from activation of mesolimbic dopamine neurons, whereas in the NACC the reinforcement may be dopamine-independent. Finally, it appears that both μ and δ, but not κ, opioid receptors may mediate the positive reinforcing actions of opioid compounds.

A Link Between Motor Stimulation
and Positive Reinforcement?

As noted above, studies have demonstrated that dopamine release in the NACC is responsible not only for the positive reinforcing actions of psychomotor stimulants (see above) but also for the motor activation produced by these compounds. Administration of psychomotor stimulants into the NACC, but not into other dopamine terminal regions, elicits motor activation (56). In addition, lesions of dopamine terminals in this nucleus interfere with the motor activating effects of psychomotor stimulants (57). Significantly, this nucleus appears to also mediate both positive reinforcing (see above) and motor activating effects of opioid compounds (126–128). The motor activating effects of opioids in the NACC are dopamine-independent (126–128). The association between positive reinforcement and motor activation has been recognized by several investigators (28,128–132) and has recently been the subject of a global theory of addiction (133). The central thesis of this theory, proposed by Wise and Bozarth, is that a common biological mechanism mediates the motor activating and positive reinforcing properties of self-administered drugs. At first, this theory might seem counterintuitive; many self-administered drugs, including opioids, barbituates, and benzodiazepines, have motor depressant actions when injected systemically. However, when examined more closely, these drugs appear to have biphasic effects on locomotion, with stimulant properties at low doses and depressant actions at higher doses (133). In the case of opioids, the locomotor activating properties have been localized to the NACC, whereas the motor depressant actions have been localized to the periaqueductal gray region (126,127,134). The apparent contradiction to the theory may therefore be attributed to motor depressant side effects of the drug; actions at a distant site may mask the behavioral **expression** of the associated motor stimulation without interfering with reinforcement. This would suggest that although the systems mediating motor stimulation and reinforcement may be the same, there is not an obligatory link between reinforcement and the behavioral expression of motor activation. Indeed, studies have found that the motor activating effect of psychomotor stimulants may sometimes be prevented without interfering with their reinforcing actions (37, 135).

Although it is still widely untested, this theory provides an interesting framework with which to examine self-administered drugs. One could take advantage of the association between motor activation and reinforcement by looking to previous research on one aspect of the pair in attempting to understand the other. For example, one might examine the results of studies on the locomotor activating properties of self-administered drugs when attempting to plan studies or draw conclusions about their reinforcing actions. Studies on the motor stimulating effects of both opioids and psychomotor stimulants suggests that the ventral pallidum is the primary output pathway from the NACC for expression of this behavior (131). If the association between motor activation and reinforcement is indeed valid, then one would predict that the ventral pallidum would also be important to the positive reinforcing actions of both opioids and psychomotor stimulants. In addition, the above-noted observation that the locomotor activating effect of opioids in the NACC are dopamine-independent is consistent with our suggestion that the reinforcing actions of opioids in this nucleus may be independent of dopamine. The association between motor stimulation and positive reinforcement may provide a valuable tool with which to understand the brain systems that mediate each of these behavioral functions.

The Nucleus Accumbens and Positive Reinforcement

The NACC and the MPC are among the major terminal regions for dopamine cell bodies located in the VTA, or A10 cell group. This system of projections, sometimes referred to as the mesolimbic, mesocortical, or mesocorticolimbic dopamine pathway, appears to play an important gating role in limbic-emotional function. The NACC, in particular, which receives input from traditional limbic cortices such as MPC, hippocampus, and amygdala, and sends outputs to pallidal motor pathways (see below), has been termed a limbic-motor interface, whereby emotions are translated into motor actions (136,137). The mesolimbic dopamine projection to the NACC is in an excellent position to modulate this interface and to bias the ability of motivational-emotional signals to gain access to motor output. Indeed, recent work has found that mesolimbic dopamine can modulate the ability of signals from the amygdala to affect neurons in the NACC and in the ventral pallidal NACC output (138–140). This theory fits well with a role for the NACC in the positive reinforcing actions of psychomotor stimulant drugs. It would appear that these drugs may produce their reinforcing effects by artificially activating a "dopamine amplification system that enhances those positive affective states prevailing in the organism at a given time" (29), allowing the positive emotional states to gain access to motor output pathways. Likewise, opioid receptors located on postsynaptic neurons in the NACC, or on presynaptic nerve terminals of limbic inputs to this nucleus, could produce a similar amplification of positive affect, allowing neural communications signaling positive emotional states access to the motor output system. The theory that the NACC may serve as a limbic-motor interface is strongly consistent with the aforementioned association between motor activation and positive reinforcement function. Additionally, as discussed below, the NACC may be an important interface between limbic and "visceromotor" output. Although the significance of this visceral link is currently unclear, it is interesting to speculate that perhaps visceral associations of reinforcement may be involved in the self-administration of drugs.

To summarize, the research outlined above on psychomotor stimulants and opioid compounds has identified four brain sites important to the positive reinforcing actions of these drugs: the MPC, the NACC, the LH, and the VTA. The question is then raised as to whether these brain sites are independently involved in reinforcement or are perhaps part of a neural "reinforcement circuit." In fact, independent neuroanatomical research has identified a circuit loop that contains within it each of these sites, with suggestions that this circuit may play an important role in reinforcement function (141). Thus, the MPC, the NACC, the LH, and the VTA are intimately associated components of a recognized circuit. We will refer to this circuit as the "limbic-motor reinforcement circuit" (Figure 2.6). This nomenclature refers to the fact that both limbic-related and motor-related brain pathways are involved in the circuitry, and also

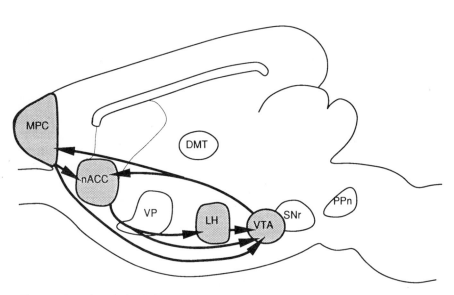

FIGURE 2.6. Saggital rab brain section illustrating the "limbic-motor reinforcement circuit." Arrows represent demonstrated pathways directly connecting the four brain sites involved in opioid and psychomotor stimulant reinforcement to each other (shaded regions). Unshaded regions represent the motor outputs from the circuit. Limbic inputs to the circuit are not shown. DMT = dorsomedial nucleus of the thalamus; LH = lateral hypothalamus; MPC = medial prefrontal cortex; nACC = nucleus accumbens; PPn = pedunculopontine nucleus; SNr = substantia nigra pars reticulata; VP = ventral pallidum; VTA = ventral tegmental area.

to the above-noted association between reinforcing and motor activating effects of drugs that act on this circuitry. The recognition that these sites are intimately interconnected provides a new vantage point from which to study the neuroanatomy of positive reinforcement and drug self-administration. In the next section we will examine in detail some important components of the limbic-motor reinforcement circuit, paying particular attention to the chemical neuroanatomy. This examination will help us to gain an understanding of the ways in which self-administered drugs access this circuitry to produce their positive reinforcing actions.

The Limbic-Motor Reinforcement Circuit

The body of behavioral and pharmacological work summarized above suggest that the VTA, NACC, LH, and MPC play prominent roles in drug reinforcement. However, the complexity of interplay between the aforementioned brain loci and other brain structures dictates careful consideration of the anatomical context in which these systems operate. Therefore, in this section we will examine, in some detail, the nature and uniqueness of the VTA to NACC projection, the pathway studied most extensively in relation to the self-administration of drugs; we will discuss the input-output relationships of these brain sites, with particular attention paid to connectivity with limbic and motor systems; and lastly, we will focus on the organization of opioid peptide systems believed to play an essential role in reinforcement, motor behavior, and self-administration.

The VTA-NACC Connection

The dopamine innervation of the NACC is derived primarily from the A10 catecholaminergic cell group in the VTA. Minor DA inputs to NACC also emanate from the extreme medial substantia nigra pars compacta and retrorubral nucleus, particularly in regions of these nuclei in proximity to the VTA (142). Projections from the VTA provide a roughly topographic distribution of fibers into the region of the NACC, with medial cell groups projecting predominantly to ventral NACC and lateral groups projecting dorsolaterally to the remainder of the NACC and the ventral striatum. The VTA projection to the NACC exhibits an apparent continuity with innervation of the striatum derived from the adjacent substantia nigra pars compacta. The substantia nigra pars compacta distributes terminals to the striatum in a ventromedial to dorsolateral gradient, extending the DA inne᷎vation of this structural from roughly the dorsolateral border of the input from VTA (142).

Recent studies indicate that larger populations (approximately 33–50%) of VTA DA neurons projecting to the NACC contain cholecystokinin (CCK) immunoreactivity (143). Colocalization of CCK-ir (immunoreactivity) and DA within substantia nigra pars compacta neurons occurs with a considerably lesser frequency, suggesting that substantia nigra pars compacta-striatal and VTA-NACC projections are neurochemically distinct. Other reports indicate that some 10–15% of VTA CCK-ir neurons also contain neurotensin (NT)-ir; a relatively small population of VTA cells contain NT-ir alone (10%). Very few NT-ir neurons can be localized to the substantia nigra pars compacta (144). Examination of terminal fields within the NACC reveals that tyrosine hydroxylase (TH) positive fibers (i.e., dopamine fibers) are distributed throughout the NACC, exhibiting densest staining in the medial region of the nucleus. Both CCK-ir and NT-ir appear to be largely confined to this medial, TH-rich region of NACC (143,145,146). These reports strongly indicate a large population of VTA neurons projecting to NACC are capable of releasing a "cocktail" of neuromodulatory substances, including DA, DA and CCK, DA and NT, and DA, CCK, and NT. They also suggest an organizational "gradient" within the NACC, which will be dealt with in more detail below.

Nucleus Accumbens Connectivity

The distribution of afferents to the NACC strongly implicates this region as a interface between neostriatal and limbic systems. Some of the major afferent inputs to NACC are illustrated in Figure 2.7. In contrast to the immediately overlying caudate-putamen, which receives a massive projection from neocortical structures, the NACC receives limited cortical input emanating primarily from limbic cortices (medial prefrontal, perirhinal, entorhinal, and insular cortex) (147–151). These inputs most densely innervate lateral and caudal areas of NACC (147,150).

The hippocampus and amygdala provide characteristic patterns of innervation to the NACC. The major hippocampal inputs into NACC arise from the subiculum, prosubiculum, and to a lesser extent CA1, and terminate primarily near the medial border of the nucleus (147,148,150–153). In contrast, projections from the amygdala, arising chiefly from the basolateral and basomedial nuclei, innervate the entire NACC and are particularly dense at the caudal and lateral extent of the nucleus (147,152,154,155). Unlike hippocampal input, the amygdala innervation is not NACC-specific; basolateral-basomedial amygdala innervates a large extent of the ventral striatum and olfactory tubercle (155). Retrograde transport of tritiated aspartate indicates that a portion of the input to NACC from amygdala may utilize glutamate or aspartate as a neurotransmitter-neuromodulator (156). Some immunochemical data suggest that the amygdala (and possibly prefrontal cortex) may in addition provide a substantial portion (60%) of the CCk input into NACC (in particular, the lateral portion of this nucleus) and the striatum (150). However, it should be noted that other studies indicate a disappearance of CCK-ir fibers in NACC following 6-OHDA lesions of the VTA and hypothalamic transections, particularly in areas of CCK-TH colocalization (143). Additional projections to the NACC are derived from

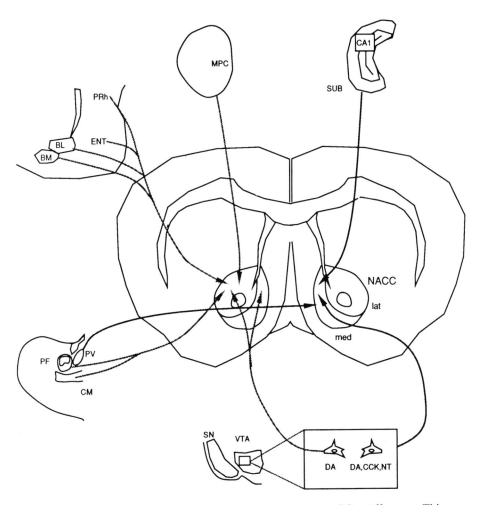

FIGURE 2.7. Connectivity of the nucleus accumbens (NACC): Afferents. This illustration depicts some of the major afferents to the NACC as described in the literature. Input from the medial prefrontal (MPC), entorhinal (ENT), and perirhinal (PRh) cortices project predominantly to the lateral and caudal regions of the NACC. Input from the basolateral (BL) and basomedial (BM) amygdala also heavily innervate this region of NACC. Thalamic inputs manifest a topographical innervation of NACC; the thalamic parafascicular (PFT) and centromedial (CM) innervate the lateral NACC; the paraventricular nucleus (PVT), in particular its dorsal portion, innervates medial regions of the NACC. Afferents from the hippocampal formation, arising from subfield CA1 and the subiculum (SUB), project primarily to the medial NACC. The VTA provides a somewhat heterogeneous input into the NACC. Dopamine (DA)-positive fibers from the VTA innervate the entire NACC, as well as a substantial portion of the ventral striatum and olfactory tubercle. A particularly heavy DA innervation may be observed in the medial NACC. However, some DA neurons in the VTA also synthesize cholecystokinin (CCK) and/or neurotensin (NT); these multiple-transmitter neurons appear to project predominantly to the medial NACC, corresponding to the area of densest DA innervation. See text Table 2.2 for further details. SN = substantia nigra.

forebrain, thalamic, and brainstem loci and are summarized in Table 2.2. It should be noted that the majority of these input are either considered part of, or are connected with, the limbic system (eg, bed nucleus of the stria terminalis, midline thalamic nuclei).

The major efferent projections of NACC neurons are summarized in Table 2.2. Efferent outflow of the NACC appears to be, to some degree, organized into limbic and somatic motor compartments (see Figure 2.8). Efferents from the medial region of NACC project heavily to the ventral pallidum and to LH; additional efferents terminate in the bed nucleus of the stria terminalis, lateral septum, medial preoptic area, VTA, retroru-bral nucelus, the central gray, and the pedunculopontine tegmental nucleus (157–160). All of the above structures have been included in, or associated with, the limbic system. The lateral region of NACC, on the

TABLE 2.2 Major connection of the nucleus accumbens (NACC)

Afferent origin	Primary terminal localization in NACC
1. Telencephalon	
Prefrontal cortex	Lateral
Suprarhinal cortex	Lateral
Perirhinal cortex	Lateral
Entorhinal cortex	Ventromedial
Hippocampal formation:	Medial
CA1, subiculum	
Basolateral, basomedial	Whole nucleus; densest posterolateral
amygdala	
2. Diencephalon	
Thalamus:	
centromedial	Lateral
paraventricular:	
dorsal	Dorsomedial
ventral	Ventrolateral
parafascicular	Lateral
reuniens	Central
rhomboidues	Central
Hypothalamus/preoptic area:	
lateral hypothalamus	Not specified (scattered)
preoptic area	Not specified (scattered)
3. Mesencephalon	
Ventral tegmental area:	Whole nucleus
interfascicular nucleus	Ventromedial
paranigral nucleus	Medial
parabrachial pigmented nucleus	Ventrolateral
Substantia nigra:	
extreme medial pars compacta	Not specified
Dorsal Raphe	Not specified
4. Rhombencephalon	
Parabrachial	Not specified
Locus coeruleus	Not specified
Nucleus of the solitary tract	Not specified
Ventrolateral medulla	Not specified

TABLE 2.2 (*Continued*)

Efferent target	Primary origin in NACC
1. Telencephalon	
Lateral septum	Medial
Bed nucleus of the stria terminalis	Medial
Ventral pallidum	Medial (densest) and lateral
Subcommissural globus pallidus	Lateral (densest) and medial
2. Diencephalon	
Thalamus:	
paratenial	Medial
mediodorsal	Medial
lateral habenuia	Medial
Hypothalamus:	
lateral hypothalamus	Medial
Medial preoptic area	Medial
Lateral preoptic area	Medial
Entopeduncular nucleus	Lateral
3. Mesencephalon	
Ventral tegmental area	Medial
Substantia nigra:	
pars compacta	Lateral
pars reticulata	Lateral
Pedunculopontine nucleus	Medial
Central gray	Medial

This table is an attempted synthesis of several literature reports (146–160).

other hand, projects to structures associated with the extrapyramidal motor system, including the ventral pallidum, subcommissural globus pallidus, entopeduncular nucleus, substantia nigra pars reticulata, and retrorubal nucleus, and as such possesses an output organization similar to that of the neostriatum (157).

Electrophysiological and pharmacological studies (161,162) suggest that the projection from NACC to ventral pallidum utilizes γ-aminobutyric acid (GABA) as a neurotransmitter and can hence be associated with inhibitory influences on pallidal cells. A GABA innervation of the VTA by NACC projection neurons is indicated by immunohistochemical data (163). Colocalization studies indicate that projection neurons of the NACC may contain NT, enkephalin (ENK), GABA, substance P, dynorphin or any combination of the above to varying degrees; following hypothalamic hemitransections, NT, ENK, substance P, and GABA immunoreactivity in the VTA, substantia nigra, and retrorubral nucleus were substantially reduced on the side of the transection (164).

VTA Connectivity

The connectivity of the VTA has been studied extensively; one is referred to the recent view of Oades and Halliday (165) for in-depth neuroanatomical analysis of this region. Efferent connections of this region are fairly

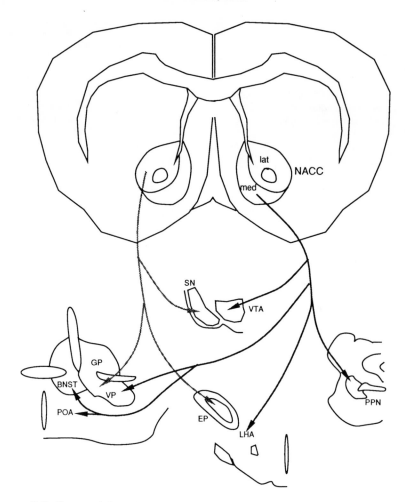

FIGURE 2.8. Connectivity of the nucleus accumbens (NACC): Efferents. Some major projections of the NACC, dervied from literature reports, are depicted in this illustration. The lateral region of the NACC appears to project to primarily extrapyramidal motor structures. Major outputs include the ventral pallidum (VP) and subcommissural globus pallidus (GP), the substantia nigra pars reticulata (SN), and the entopeduncular nucleus. The medial region, on the other hand, appears to connect with limbic brain regions, including the ventral tegmental area (VTA), bed nucleus of the stria terminalis (BNST), preoptic area (POA), and lateral hypothalamus (LHA), as well as the VP and pedunculopontine nucleus (PPN). The medial-lateral distinctions drawn here are based on density of outputs; some degree of overlap exists in these projection sytems. See text and Table 2.2 for further details.

well characterized, forming the "mesolimbic" dopamine system. This system has historically been defined on the basis of its dopamine content; however, a study by Swanson (166) clearly shows that this criterion may be an oversimplification (see below). Numerous reports have demonstrated that the VTA projects dopamine neurons to limbic cortices (entorhinal, cingulate, suprahinal, insular, and prefrontal); see Fallon and Loughlin (141) for review. Subcortical telencephalic innervation is supplied to amygdaloid nuclei (central, medial, lateral), the lateral septum, substantia innominata, olfactory nuclei, and olfactory tubercle, as well as the ventral striatum and NACC, as discussed above (165).

Double-labeling experiments have convincingly demonstrated that projection systems of the VTA are heterogeneous in their content of DA. For instance, VTA projections to the NACC and lateral suptum contain a very high percentage of TH-positive cells (85% and 72%, respectively). VTA innervation of amygdala and entorhinal cortex were 53% and 46% dopaminergic, whereas only 30% of VTA neurons projecting to suprarhinal and prefrontal cortices contained DA. Less than 10% of VTA neurons projecting to hippocampus, lateral habenula, and locus coeruleus were DA-containing (166). This important study illustrates that the projection system of the VTA is more than a solely dopaminergic system and implies that this nucleus contributes different sorts of information to different brain regions.

Consideration of major afferents to the VTA yields valuable insight into the importance of this cell group. VTA receives dense innervation from the NACC, bed nucleus of the stria terminalis, nucleus of the diagonal band, ventral pallidum, lateral preoptic area, and LH in the tel- and diencephalon. Considerable input is received from prefrontal and suprarhinal cortex, olfactory tubercle, amygdala, and lateral habenula as well (160,165,167,168). The outstanding common characteristic of these projections to VTA is the fact that all of the above structures are in receipt of VTA efferents and thus show an astounding degree of connectional reciprocity.

On the basis of connectivity of the VTA, it is evident that this region is in receipt of highly integrated input (entorhinal and prefrontal cortical projections), input from limbic regions involved in motivational-emotional function (amygdala, LH), and input from regions known to provide wide-reaching innervation to large segments of the cerebrum (locus coeruleus, Raphe nuclei). Through reciprocal connections with these brain structures the VTA is in a position to provide information to these diverse regions as well.

Other Reinforcement Loci

Additional brain regions strongly associated with drug self-administration and reinforcement include the prefrontal cortex and LH. Full discussion of the input and outputs of these regions are beyond the scope of this chapter, however, it is of particular interest to note that these nuclei are in a position to interact monosynaptically with the VTA and NACC. The LH, for instance, receives a direct input from the "limbic" NACC (157), and supplies innervation to the VTA (167,169). The prefrontal cortex receives a dense innervation from the VTA (141), and in turn projects to NACC (147–150) and VTA (167). Thus, these additional "reinforcement loci" both receive afferents from the project afferents to the VTA-NACC pathway. The connections among these four brain sites makes it evident that they are intimately-related components of an easily identifiable circuit loop (141), what we are calling the "limbic-motor reinforcement circuit." The abundance of evidence demonstrating that the individual sites within the circuit are involved in reinforcement suggests that the circuit as a whole may be important both in the self-administration of drugs and in brain mechanisms of reinforcement.

Opioid Peptide and Receptor Distribution in Reinforcement Circuits

The obvious importance of opioids in reinforcement processes indicates that opioid peptides should be localized in brain regions critical for expression of behavioral indices of reinforcement. To explore this issue with some detail, we have prepared sections stained for peptides derived from the three defined opioid peptide systems and for the catecholaminergic synthetic enzyme TH. Opioid antibodies were directed against leu-enkephalin (ENK) (PROENK system), dynorphin 1-17 (DYN) (PRO-DYN system), and β-endorphin (POMC) (proopiomelanocrotin system) peptides. Results are indicated in Figures 2.9 to 2.15.

Opioid peptide innervation of NACC is derived from all three opioid precursor systems. A schematic summary of opioid innervation of this area is illustrated on the left side of Figure 2.9; immunostained sections stained for TH (Figure 2.10A), and opioid peptides (Figures 2.10B–D) are also presented. Both ENK- and DYN-positive fibers densely innervate the ventromedial aspect of NACC (Figures 2.10B, C). Indeed, examination of adjacent sections suggests considerable overlap of ENK and DYN fiber networks in the ventromedial NACC. The dorsal and lateral regions of the NACC are more sparsely innervated by ENK- and DYN-positive fibers (Figure 2.9). ENK fibers present in the dorsal and lateral NACC tend to be clumped into patchlike aggregations. POMC fibers appear to be distributed throughout the NACC, in accordance with our previous findings (170). Although the POMC fiber density is generally light, the medial aspect of NACC, particularly the region just ventromedial to the anterior commissure, appears to contain the heaviest fiber staining (Figure 2.10D). Examination of adjacent sections stained for TH (eg, Figure 2.10A) illustrates that the area of densest ENK and DYN staining by and large overlaps the region of densest DA innervation, although

Opioid Peptide Terminals   *Opioid Receptors*

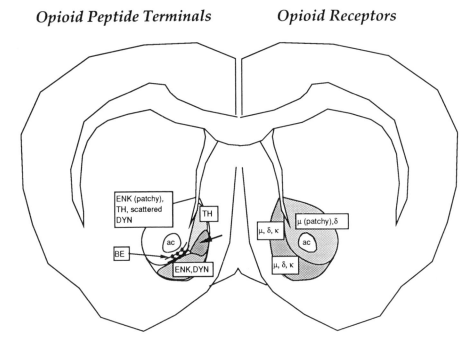

FIGURE 2.9. Schematic summary of opioid peptide-containing and tyrosine hydroxylase (TH)–containing fibers (left) and opioid receptor binding (right) in the NACC. Fibers staining positively for enkephalin (ENK) (proenkephalin system) and dynorphin (DYN) (prodynorphin system) form dense aggregations in the ventromedial NACC. The ENK- and DYN-rich region of the NACC shows a substantial but incomplete overlap with the region of richest TH innervation (see arrow). ENK-positive fibers are also present in the dorsal and lateral NACC, tending to form patchlike aggregations; scattered DYN fibers can also be observed in these regions. β-Endorphin-positive fibers (proopiomelanocortin system) can be localized to the medial NACC; these fibers tend to be densest in regions just ventral and medial to the anterior commissure (ac) (beaded fibers on illustration). Receptor autoradiographs reveal dense binding of δ-, κ-, μ-receptor-specific opioid ligands in NACC. Whereas δ binding is quite heavy throughout the nucleus, μ binding exhibits a patchy pattern throughout the NACC but is particularly dense in the medial region; κ binding is particularly dense in the medial NACC.

considerable numbers of ENK and DYN fibers occupy the region immediately ventral to this area (Figure 2.10B and C). The TH-rich region corresponds to areas receiving the greatest density of CCK and NT fibers (143,145), and to the region in receipt of fibers from the hippocampal formation.

Cell bodies positive for ENK and DYN can be localized to the NACC (presented schematically in Figure 2.11). ENK-positive neurons are seen

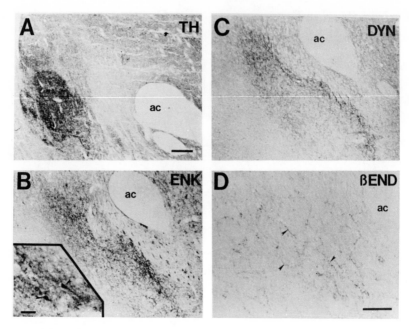

FIGURE 2.10. Photomicrographs of immunostained sections through the NACC reacted with antisera directed against (A) tyrosine hydroxylase (TH), (B) leu-enkephalin (ENK), (C) dynorphin 1-17 (DYN), and (D) β-endorphin (βEND). A. Stain for TH shows dense innervation of the medial NACC. Fiber density is particularly pronounced in the dorsomedial aspect of the nucleus at this level. ac = anterior commissure. Bar = 100 μm. B. Stain for ENK. A dense aggregation of ENK-positive fibers can be observed at the ventromedial border of the NACC near the NACC-ventral pallidum junction; contrast with patchy appearance of staining seen caudolateral to the anterior commissure (ac) in this section. Note partial overlap with the area of dense TH staining in A; same magnification as in A. Inset depicts ENK-positive cell bodies localized to this region. Bar = 20 μm. C. Stain for DYN. DYN fibers can also be localized preferentially to the ventromedial border of the NACC, overlapping the ENK innervation of this region seen on a neighboring section (B). The DYN innervation of NACC partially overlaps the region of densest TH staining in the medial NACC. Same magnification as in A. D. Stain for βEND. High-power view of scattered βEND-containing fibers in the proximity of the ac. Bar = 40 μm.

predominantly in the ventromedial NACC (Figure 2.10B inset; see also 171). The ability of neurons in the NACC to synthesize ENK is further corroborated by localization of PROENK messenger RNA to cells in the NACC *in situ* hybridization histochemistry; indeed, the number of cells positive for PROENK mRNA appears to eclipse that observed by immunohistochemistry (172). DYN-positive cells are more evenly distributed in the nucleus than are ENK neurons, with a tendency to aggregate in the medial region (Figure 2.11) (171). No POMC-positive cell bodies are seen in the NACC, in accordance with previous data (170). Although these studies indicate the presence of DYN and ENK (but not POMC) in NACC cell bodies, the role of DYN and ENK neurons within this nucleus remains to be definitively determined. Studies reported to date do not adequately address whether these neurons act as local-circuit or projection neurons or both.

POMC peptide innervation of the NACC is believed to originate in POMC-producing cells in the arcuate nucleus of the hypothalamus (170). Origins of proenkephalin and prodynorphin peptide innervation of the NACC are more difficult to specify; no studies have been designed specifically to address this issue to date. Among the known afferent systems to the NACC, the bed nucleus of the stria terminalis and preoptic area contain appreciable aggregations of opioid peptide cell bodies (171,173). However, the localization of ENK- and DYN-positive cell bodies in the NACC and surrounding regions clearly raises the possibility that ENK and DYN innervation of this structure arises partially or wholly from local-circuit neurons.

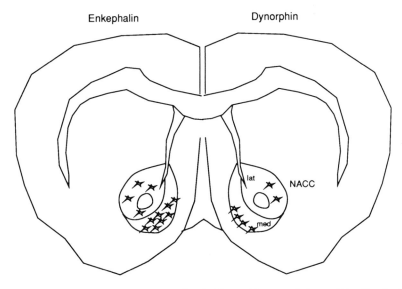

FIGURE 2.11. Schematic summary of opioid peptide-containing cell bodies in the NACC, based on our stained material and on literature reports (see 'text). ENK-positive cells bodies (proenkephalin system) are present in limited quantities throughout the nucleus (left side of diagram); the greatest density of ENK cells corresponds to the region of densest ENK fiber staining in the ventromedial NACC. DYN-positive cells (prodynorphin system) are also scattered throughout the nucleus; the greatest number of cell bodies are seen in the ventromedial NACC. In general, the number of ENK-positive cells exceeds the number of DYN-positive cells in all regions of the NACC.

Opiate receptor autoradiography reveals that μ-, δ-, and κ-ligands all bind in the region of the rat NACC. Digitized images derived from receptor autoradiographs are presented in Figures 2.12A–C; a schematic representation is included in Figure 2.9. The distribution of binding is quite heterogeneous among the receptor subtypes examined. As shown in Figure 2.12A, δ-receptor binding is quite dense throughout the extent of

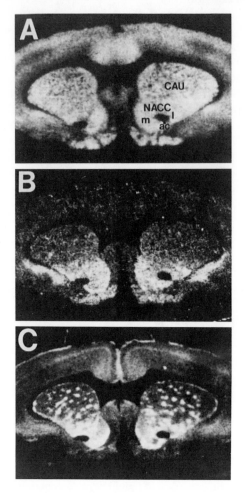

FIGURE 2.12. Digitized images of receptor autoradiographs through the level of the NACC in the rat. *A*. Delta binding, which is quite dense throughout both the NACC and caudate nucleus (CAU) at this rostrocaudal level. No obvious differences in binding density can be observed between the medial (m) and lateral (1) NACC. *B*. Kappa binding. Dense κ-binding can be observed in the medial region of the NACC, standing in marked contrast to binding in the remainder of the NACC and the overlying caudate nucleus (CAU). *C*. Mu binding, which is quite dense throughout the NACC. In the lateral region of this, μ-binding exhibits a patchy appearance qualitatively similar to that seen in the caudate.

the NACC. In contrast, κ-receptor binding is found predominantly in the medial extent of NACC (Figure 2.12*B*), the region that receives hippocampal afferents and DA, CCK, NT-positive fibers and contains the greatest density of ENK- and DYN-staining. Although μ-binding represents a patchy but quite dense distribution throughout the entire NACC, in general the medial NACC retains relatively high levels of μ-binding (Figure 2.12*C*). The patchy nature of μ-binding in the remainder of NACC strongly resembles that of the overlying caudate-putamen. It should be noted that in comparison to other brain regions, the density of binding for all three receptor types is quite high (174,175).

The VTA, while being a region responsive to reinforcing effects of opioid peptides, receives a relatively modest opioid input. The distribution of TH and opioid peptide cell bodies and fibers are summarized schematically in Figure 2.13; representative immunostained sections are shown in Figure 2.14*A–C*. Our stains for ENK, DYN, and POMC (not shown) reveal an intermediate density of fibers localized throughout the VTA (Figures 2.13 and 2.14*B,C*). ENK staining is somewhat denser than that of DYN or POMC (Figure 2.14*B*). In contrast, DYN-positive fibers densely innervate the neighboring substantia nigra pars compacta and pars reticulata (Figure 2.14*C*). The VTA, though replete with TH-positive perikarya (Figure 2.14*A*), is largely devoid of DYN and POMC cell bodies; a modest number of ENK-positive perikarya can be localized by immunohistochemical and *in situ* hybridization methods (172,173). Nuclei in proximity to the VTA contain numerous ENK- and DYN-containing neurons; among these, the interpeduncular nucleus is heavily populated by ENK cell bodies, whereas the lateral substantia nigra pars compacta and the midbrain Raphe nuclei contain considerable numbers of both ENK- and DYN-positive cells (171,173). Whether these neighboring regions contribute opioid innervation of the VTA remains to be determined. Some additional evidence suggests that at least part of the opioid peptide innervation of the VTA may come from distal sites. Combined retrograde tracing and immunocytochemical studies indicate that the VTA may receive a DYN projection from the LH (176). Unilateral midbrain transections cause a depletion of ENK staining in the VTA and substantia nigra pars reticulata, suggesting that telencephalic ENK neurons may innervate this region (164).

Among the three opioid receptor types the μ-type shows the heaviest binding in receptor autoradiographs of the VTA (Figures 2.13 and 2.15); see also Mansour et al (174). A modest amount of κ binding is also detectable in this region; delta receptor binding, however, does not exceed background. It should be noted that, in comparison with other brain regions in rat, binding of all three receptor types is quite low (174).

The LH contains large numbers of scattered DYN and ENK cells (171,173), and is innervated by fibers specific for all three opioid precursors (170,171,173). Opiate receptor binding for the three known receptor types is rather sparse; there is evidence for limited κ binding and

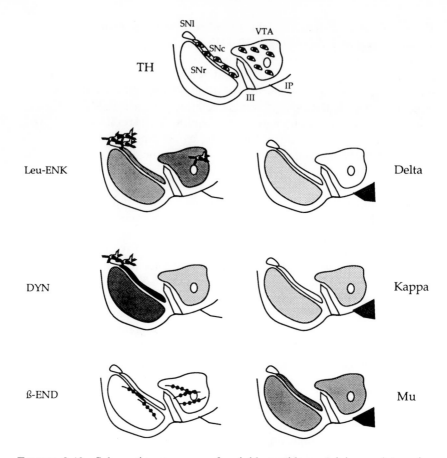

FIGURE 2.13. Schematic summary of opioid peptide-containing and tyrosine dydroxylase (TH)–containing fibers (left) and opioid receptor binding (right) in the ventral tegmental area (VTA) and substantia nigra (SN) of the rat. Intensity of shading in relevant areas is proportional (qualitatively) to intensity of opioid peptide fiber staining. Densely packed aggregations of TH-positive cell bodies are observed in the VTA and substantia nigra pars compacta (SNc), forming the mesolimbic and nigrostriatal dopaminergic pathways, respectively. Enkephalin (ENK)-positive fibers (proenkephalin system) modestly innervate the VTA and SNc and SNr (pars reticulata). Scattered ENK cell bodies can be localized in the lateral SN (SN1). Dynorphin (DYN)-positive fibers (prodynorphin system) densely innervate the SNc and SNr; in contrast, the VTA receives a quite limited DYN input. Cell bodies are present in limited quantities in the SN1. Fibers derived from the proopiomelanocortin (POMC) system are present in limited quantities throughout the VTA and SN. Levels of opioid receptor binding in the VTA (and SN) are generally low. Some degree of μ binding can be observed in the VTA; slightly higher levels of binding can be seen in the SNr. Kappa binding is quite limited in the VTA and SN of the rat, whereas δ binding does not exceed background in this species. It should be noted that considerable species variation exists in opioid receptor binding in these regions (174,175).

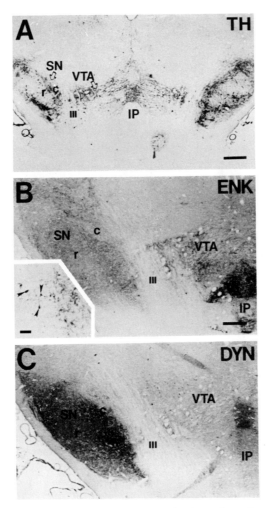

FIGURE 2.14. Photomicrographs of immunostained sections through the ventral tegmental area (VTA) and substantia nigra (SN) of the rat, stained for (A) tyrosine hydroxylase (TH), (B) leu-enkephalin (ENK), and (C) dynorphin 1-17 (DYN). A. TH staining is a low-power photomicrograph of the VTA and SN, depicting TH cell bodies and fibers in the VTA and SN pars compacta (c). Bar = 500 μm. III = third nerve, IP = interpeduncular nucleus. B. Higher-power view of ENK staining in this region. ENK-positive fibers relatively lightly innervate the VTA and SNc and pars reticulata (r) at this level. ENK cell bodies can be observed in the neighboring IP; scattered ENK cells can also be seen in the VTA itself (inset). Bar = 200 μm. C. DYN stain in VTA/SN region. DYN-positive fibers densely innervate the SNc and r. In contrast, few DYN fibers are localized in the VTA proper. Same magnification as in B.

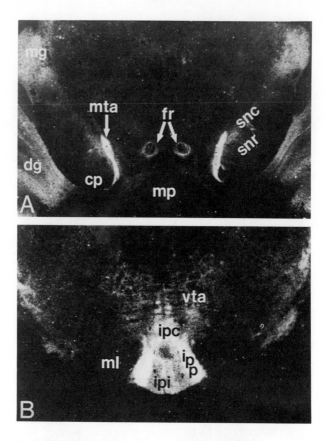

FIGURE 2.15. Photomicrographs of emulsion-dipped sections through the SN/
VTA, depicting μ-receptor binding in this region. Moderate levels of μ binding
can be observed in both (A) the SN, and (B) the VTA of the rat. A. Substantia
nigra. Mu binding is evident in the substantia nigra pars compacts (snc) and to a
more limited exetnt in pars reticulata (snr). dg = dentate gyrus, mta = medial
terminal nucleus, accessory optic tract, cp = cerebral peduncle, fr = fasciculus
retroflexus; mp = mammillary peduncle. B. VTA, mesencephalon-pontine junction. Mu binding is evidenct in the VTA; heavy binding is observed in the
subjacent interpeduncular complex (ipc = interpeduncular nucleus, central, ipi =
interpeduncular nucleus, inner posterior subnucleus, ipp = interpeduncular
nucleus, paramedian, and ml = medial lemniscus). Little κ and δ binding is
observed in the SN or VTA (see text and Figure 2.13).

a small amount of μ binding. As indicated above, DYN-positive neurons
appear to project from LH to the VTA (176).

Prefrontal cortex contains a limited number of DYN- and ENK-positive
fibers and cell bodies, which do not distinguish it from other cortical
regions (171,173). Binding of μ-, κ-, δ-receptors is present in this region; μ
binding is particularly dense relative to the other subtypes (see 174).

Synthesis: Opioid Peptides in Reinforcement Circuitry

What can we conclude regarding the position of opioids in circuits mediating drug self-administration and reinforcement, based on the connectional-neurochemical data summarized above? First, opioid peptide-containing fibers densely innervate the medial and ventromedial region of the NACC, overlapping the region of the densest TH fiber staining and the region reported to contain appreciable CCK- and NT-immunoreactivity (143,145). Opioid peptides are thus in a position to directly interact with integration of VTA afferents and NACC projection neurons. As discussed above, neuropharmacological evidence clearly suggests that DA and opioids may act at the level of the NACC, perhaps mediating the positive reinforcing properties of opioid compounds and psychomotor stimulants. Second, preferential localization of large aggregations of κ-, δ-, and μ-receptors at the level of the medial NACC suggests that each of the three receptor types may be involved in opioid integratory processes in this region. The overlap between the region of highest *opioid receptor density,* highest density of *POMC, DYN, and ENK fibers,* highest density of *TH, CCK, and NT fibers* and projections from *hippocampus and subiculum* in the *medial* NACC indicate that this particular subdivision of NACC may play a particularly important role in integration of limbic input–NACC output. Finally, evidence suggests that the *medial* NACC projects primarily to limbic sites (157). Projections to the lateral hypothalamic area place NACC outflow in a position to influence hypothalamic "motor" outflow, including neuroendocrine secretions via interactions with median eminence-projecting and posterior pituitary-projecting neurons, and autonomic activity via interactions with brainstem and spinal cord sympathetic and parasympathetic nuclei (177). The importance of this NACC-LH connection should not be underestimated; the connection of the NACC with both somatic motor (via the ventral pallidum and subcommissural globus pallidus) and hypothalamic outflow indicates that the NACC is capable of integrating both somatic- and visceral-motor functions.

Further evidence suggesting opioid involvement in visceromotor activity stems from the strong opioid presence in the lateral hypothalamic area. Considerable numbers of DYN- and ENK-positive cell bodies are observed in this area, as are DYN and ENK fibers. A DYN projection from this region to the VTA has been reported (176). Thus lateral hypothalamic opioid peptide cells are in a position to process or relay NACC information to both endocrine and autonomic "motor" cells and to cells spreading VTA innervation to the mesolimbic system.

Opiate integration in the VTA appears to be mediated by relatively few opioid-positive fibers and receptors as compared with the density of these peptides in the NACC. However, as discussed above, the ability of opioids to interact with VTA function is well documented in neuropharmacological studies. It is thus possible that the relatively limited endogenous opioid peptide input to the VTA has an ability to exert a profound influence on ongoing VTA neuronal activity. In this regard, it would be of particular interest to determine whether opioid peptide fibers interact with any definable subset of VTA projection neurons and thus have a direct "channel" into a given VTA projection system.

As discussed above, knowledge of the connectional anatomy of reinforcement systems and the opioid innervation and receptor localization in these systems leads us to speculate that one potential role for opioids in this system may be integration of limbic information with somatic and particularly visceral motor control. This speculation is based on the anatomical context in which opioid peptides and receptors are placed in the NACC, VTA, and LH. Identification of specific opioid peptide systems interacting with these structures is a bit more problematic. In the NACC, exogenous opioids exhibit reinforcing properties and support drug self-administration, as discussed earlier. Actions of endogenous opioid peptides may be exerted via local circuit neurons (DYN, ENK) indigenous to the NACC or by projection neurons from hypothalamic (eg, preoptic area) or telencephalic (eg, bed nucleus of the stria terminalis) sites. Opioid peptide actions may thus be either presynaptic or postsynaptic to DA projections from the VTA and/or limbic inputs into the medial NACC.

In the VTA, opiate fibers may arise from a myriad of different sources, the most compelling of which are DYN and ENK neurons of the LH and POMC neurons of the arcuate nucleus. DYN- and ENK-positive fibers can be seen entering the region of the VTA dorsally from the midbrain Raphe nuclei, suggesting that at least some opioid innervation may be derived from this region. In addition to opioid peptide innervation from distant sources, DYN- and ENK-positive cells are observed in the lateral substantia nigra, and ENK cells in the VTA itself and the interpeduncular complex immediately adjacent to the VTA, indicating the possibility of local projections onto VTA neurons. Finally, projection neurons from the NACC may contain ENK and DYN and interact directly with VTA projection neurons. Determination of which cell groups send opioid projections to the VTA is important to analyses of reinforcement processes, in light of the positive reinforcing actions of exogenously administered opioid compounds in this region (178). Each of the above-mentioned possibilities for sources of opioid innervation of the VTA bears a different potential interpretation. For instance, opioid projections from lateral hypothalamic neurons suggest that the VTA is being apprised of or interacting with information relating to autonomic and endocrine status, in keeping with a limbic-visceromotor function of opioids in reinforcement circuits. Innervation by midbrain Raphe neurons suggests opioids may be part of a more diffuse, general system supplying information to numerous brain structures, perhaps concerning ongoing brain activity. The intriguing possibility of a direct opioid peptide projection from NACC to the VTA suggests the existence of a feedback loop in the NACC-VTA circuit, similar to that observed in the striatal-pallidal-nigrostriatal pathway (141). In such a scheme, one may postulate that the originating component of a given neuronal event (either NACC or VTA) is directly apprised of the consequences of that event.

In summary, although much is known about the chemical neuroanatomy of the sites and circuitry involved in the positive reinforcing actions of opioids and psychomotor stimulants, there is still much to learn. The identification of the limbic-motor reinforcement circuit will help by providing a focus with which to examine the neuroanatomical context of positive reinforcement and self-administration. The overlap of appropriate inputs, outputs, terminals, and receptors suggests that the medial NACC should be a site of particular research focus. If the circuitry involved in positive reinforcement is to be more fully understood, it is necessary to resolve the origin and positions of opioid peptide neurons, particularly opioid-receptive neurons of brain sites within the circuit.

Negative Reinforcing Actions of Drug Withdrawal

Although considerable recent work has examined the neural mechanisms of positive reinforcing actions of self-administered drugs, relatively little work has focused on the negative reinforcing aspects of drug withdrawal. As discussed above, however, the aversiveness of the withdrawal syndrome can contribute significantly to continued self-administration in a dependent drug user. In general, most theories of tolerance and dependence have as their central idea compensatory reactions of neuronal systems in response to chronic exposure to a drug. Upon initial exposure to a drug the acute effects (either excitation or inhibition) are completely manifest. With continued exposure, homeostatic mechanisms return the system to normal functioning despite the continued presence of drug. This is tolerance; to obtain the same magnitude of effect in a tolerant subject one must administer more drug, in addition to what is already present. Withdrawal of drug reveals the altered state of the neuronal system; without the drug to inhibit or excite the compensated system, a hyperexcitable or hypoexcitable state ensues. The withdrawal symptoms that occur, therefore, depend on the drug that was present. In the case of opioids, which acutely cause sedation in the whole animal, the withdrawal syndrome is a hyperexcitable state; in the case of psychomotor stimulants in which acute activation occurs, lethargy and depression are seen on withdrawal.

The widespread distribution of opioid receptors in mammalian tissue suggests that many sites may contribute to the opioid withdrawal syndrome. As noted by Martin (80), "contra-adaptation" to the actions of opioids takes place and "represents a complementary image of the map of the opioid depressed foci." In other words, the rebound hyperexcitability that occurs in the neurons at the opioid depressed sites following withdrawal of drug is responsible for the symptoms of abstinence. However, many of these symptoms are merely physical symptoms, contributing to the flu-like nature of withdrawal. As noted above, the anxiety and craving during withdrawal appear to be more important to continued self-administration than the physical symptoms. Are there specific sites in the CNS that might contribute to the anxiety and craving of the withdrawal syndrome?

In fact, recent research suggests that the locus coeruleus, the primary noradrenergic nucleus in the brain, may be an important site in the anxiogenic effects of opioid withdrawal. Neurons of the locus coeruleus are regulated by α_2-adrenergic autoreceptors as well as μ-opioid receptors. These receptors are both coupled to potassium channels by guanine nucleotide regulatory proteins. Activation of either receptor type by appropriate agonists will increase potassium conductance and inhibit the firing of noradrenergic neurons in this nucleus (85,86,179). Following chronic treatment with opioids these neurons become tolerant to opioid-mediated inhibition, but not α_2-mediated inhibition (180,181), in an apparent desensitization of μ-receptor coupling to the potassium channel. Upon withdrawal, these neurons display a rebound hyperexcitability (180,181), with excessive release of noradrenaline in terminal regions (182). This rebound hyperexcitability can be reversed by administration of opioids or α_2-adrenergic receptor agonists (180–182). Excessive activity of the locus coeruleus has been shown to evoke profound anxiety in experimental animals (183,184). Many of the symptoms of the opioid withdrawal syndrome, including anxiety, can be attenuated by the administration of clonidine, an α_2-receptor agonist (183,185,186). This research has led to the clinical use of clonidine in the treatment of opioid withdrawal (185,186). Interestingly, a recent study found α_2-mediated inhibition of locus coeruleus neurons by cocaine (187), raising the possibility that rebound hyperexcitability of the locus might be involved in psychomotor stimulant, as well as opioid withdrawal.

Research indicates that other sites may also be important in the manifestation of withdrawal symptoms, including the central gray region (188–191), the medial hypothalamus (24, 192), and the medial thalamus (23). The central gray region is an interesting site because of its proximity to the locus coeruleus. Considering that spread of drug following intracerebral injections may leak from caudal aspects of the central gray to the neighboring locus coeruleus, it will be of considerable interest to determine whether the central gray is indeed an independent site of opioid withdrawal. If the central gray region is found to be a distinct site for the aversive aspects of opioid withdrawal, it will be of further interest to determine whether this corresponds to the involvement of this brain region in the analgesic actions (193), or the motor depressant effects (127,134) of opioids. The possible role of the hypothalamus in opioid withdrawal is particularly intriguing because of the involvement of this brain region in homeostasis and need-based drive states. Opioids become a "need" as important as food or water to the dependent user. Perhaps the hypothalamus is involved in the profound craving of opioid withdrawal.

What about endogenous opioid peptides and receptors? What role might they play in tolerance and dependence? The discovery of the opioid peptides and receptors, not surprisingly, led to early excitement in investigators studying these properties. It was speculated that drug-induced dysregulation of opioid systems might be an important factor in the manifestation of tolerance and dependence. However, studies on opioid receptor binding were disappointing, in that no effects were seen following chronic treatment with opioids (194,195). (As noted above, it may actually be changes in the coupling of receptors to second-messenger system, rather than changes in the receptors themselves that are involved in tolerance and dependence.) Studies on enkephalins and endorphins proved equally disappointing, since no effects on brain levels of these peptides were observed following chronic opioid administration (196–199). Recent studies in our laboratory using selective antibodies for different forms of β-endorphin have confirmed the lack of effect of chronic morphine on either content or processing of β-endorphin in cell body or terminal regions of brain POMC neurons (200). Interestingly, there is preliminary evidence suggesting that messenger RNA coding for the POMC precursor may down-regulate in response to chronic morphine treatment (200,201). It is currently too early to comment on the significance of this finding; however, it does indicate a promising avenue of research.

While studies have found little effect of chronic opioids on endorphin or enkephalin peptides, recent research indicates that dynorphins may be more responsive. Preliminary studies examining brain mRNA levels PRODYN have demonstrated decreases following chronic opiate treatment (202). Paradoxically, chronic heroin (203) and chronic morphine treatment (204) appear to increase the concentration of PRODYN peptide products in various brain regions in the rat. This combination of results suggests a decrease in biosynthetic capability that is coupled with a substantial decrease in release, thereby leading to consequent accumulation of PRODYN in the neuronal stores. It is therefore possible that withdrawal-induced rebound may lead to the liberation of these accumulated peptides. In light of the κ-receptor selectivity of PRODYN peptides (see above), and the dysphoric effects of κ-receptor activation (123), these findings raise the possibility that release of dynorphins following withdrawal might play a role in withdrawal-induced dysphoria. Interestingly, recent studies indicate that repeated administration of psychomotor stimulants also causes increases in brain levels of PRODYN peptides (97,205). Moreover, the κ-selective peptides dynorphin A 1-17 and dynorphin B showed a greater relative increase than the relatively nonselective dynorphin A 1-8 (Trujillo, Day, and Akil, in preparation). Thus, long-term exposure to psychomotor stimulants and opioids causes increases in dynorphin peptide stores and may therefore permit a rebound increase in activity at dysphorigenic κ-receptor sites upon withdrawal. Although the possible relevance of these findings to the dysphoria of withdrawal are tentative, the similarities in the response of PRODYN peptides to long-term administration of opioids and psychomotor stimulants suggest that these peptides may play a role in the long-term consequences of self-administered drugs.

Future Directions

Integration: Positive and Negative Reinforcement

Whereas early theories or self-administration of drugs focused on withdrawal and negative reinforcement, more recent theories have focused on positive reinforcement. These views are not mutually exclusive. Prior to the development of physical dependence it is apparent that the positive reinforcing actions of drugs are key to their self-administration; drug taking can be stopped without aversive consequences. However, with repeated administration, opioids, psychomotor stimulants, and a number of other drugs create a state of dependence wherein absence of drug is very aversive. The physically dependent subject is therefore motivated bidirectionally to further self-administration. The positive reinforcing effect of the drug and the negative reinforcing effects of the absence of drug both contribute to self-administration in a physically dependent subject. As discussed above, it does not appear that the physical manifestations of the withdrawal syndrome are so potent that they cannot be overcome. Instead, it is the powerfully aversive emotions generated by withdrawal that appear to motivate the user to continue to self-administer. These emotions include profound anxiety and craving for the absent drug. Although not discussed above, it is also conceivable that, in a subpopulation of opiate abusers, even the initial administration is motivated by the anxiety-reducing properties of these agents. The main reinforcing value of the drug in such a case would be an antidote to negative affect rather than a search for positive affect. Whether behavior motivated in this fashion would follow a different course of chronic administration than would "pleasure seeking" behavior is ill understood. We therefore feel that it is important for researchers to study not only the positive reinforcing actions of drugs or only the negative reinforcing properties of drugs, but to combine the studies of both in order to understand more fully the factors that motivate self-administration.

The richness of the opioid systems provides an excellent opportunity to study the interplay of positive and negative reinforcement in controlling self-administration. The fact that activation of κ-receptors has been shown to be aversive to laboratory animals and dysphorigenic to humans raises some interesting possibilities. For example, since most opioid compounds interact with more than one receptor type, it is possible that the aversive consequences of κ-receptor activation compete with the rewarding properties of μ- or δ-receptor activation in self-administration of opioid compounds. This hypothesis suggests that κ-receptor blockade should increase the positive reinforcing actions of opioid drugs. Will blockade of κ-receptors, by preventing the aversive properties of opioids, increase the positive reinforcing effects of drugs such as morphine or heroin? Are κ-receptors involved in acute aversive actions of opioids, such as taste aversion? As suggested above, is the activation of κ-receptors involved in he aversiveness of withdrawal? The answers to these questions will help further to elucidate the positive reinforcing and negative reinforcing actions of opioid compounds, and the role of these properties in self-administration.

Future Strategies

What research strategies can be employed to understand the complex interplay between reinforcement, anxiety, tolerance, and dependence that contribute to the maintenance of drug-seeking behavior? Can any of the tools of modern biology help uncover the possible underlying physical reasons that lead some individuals, but not others, to seek certain drugs? These questions lie at the interface of neurobiology, psychology, and genetics, and are likely to prove quite vexing. However, we shall suggest some approaches that, though unlikely to solve them, may lead us closer to the answer, or at least to a reframing of the questions.

In general, we believe that these problems need to be attacked on three simultaneous fronts:

1. *Cell Biology*. We need a more thorough understanding of the key elements at the cellular level. This approach would involve the elucidation of the structure of the critical transmitters and receptors and the uncovering of the principles of their regulation.

2. *Circuitry*. Although some elements of the circuits are identified, the complete biochemical anatomy remains unknown. In particular, we need to describe the key nuclei and pathways, then understand the dynamics of interplay within a given circuit (eg, dopamine and opioids in reward) and across circuits (eg, positive reinforcement and negative reinforcement).

3. *The Biological Bases of Individual Differences*. Whereas rats, and even humans, may have similar cellular and anatomical organization, they express a wide behavioral range (eg, in their anxiety thresholds or their propensity toward drug seeking). Can we begin to pinpoint biological differences that govern this behavioral variation?

Cell Biology

It is now well established that opioid compounds produce their many physiological and behavioral effects by interacting with opioid receptors, mimicking the actions of endogenous opioid peptides. As outlined above, research thus far demonstrates that the μ- and δ-receptors mediate the positive reinforcing actions of opioids, whereas activation of κ-receptors is aversive.

However, these receptors remain constructs probed with pharmacological tools. We still know very little about the protein structures of opioid receptors, the coupling of these receptors to second messenger systems, or the molecular mechanisms of their up- and down-regulation. The use of molecular biological techniques will yield the nucleic acid sequences of opioid receptors and provide the starting point for the elucidation of the three-dimensional organization of these proteins, their membrane orientation, their coupling sites to G-proteins, and possible sites of posttranslational modifications, which can be critical in their regulation. In addition, cloning will finally settle the number game in opioid receptors, that is, it will determine how many types and subtypes exist in fact. It should be noted in passing that cloning of the muscarinic receptors has revealed a larger number of distinct genes than previously anticipated from pharmacological studies. This finding flew in the face of speculation that receptor subtypes are identical proteins, derived from a single gene, with differing posttranslational modifications or membrane lipid environments.

Given that the opioid receptors are to be cloned, would that facilitate our efforts to understand drug-seeking behavior? Just as the discovery of endogenous opioids did not immediately illuminate us with regard to opiate addiction, the elucidation of the opioid receptors structure is unlikely to yield immediate and dramatic insights into the mechanisms of opiate-seeking behavior. However, such findings will move us perceptibily into a more concrete realm where more basic questions can be attacked: What are the molecular mechansims of tolerance? Do opiate receptors down-regulate their numbers or decrease their affinity, despite the fact that we are currently unable to detect such changes? Or, alternatively, do they change their coupling to their associated G-protein, rendering them less efficacious, as suggested by electrophysiological studies?

While the opioid peptides' mRNA and gene structures have been elucidated, much remains to be done towards a complete understanding of their regulation from gene expression to secretion. Why so many different opioids? Why multiple copies within a vesicle? Why are highly active and selective products such as dynorphin A 1-17 converted intracellularly to less stable and less selective derivatives (dyn A 1-8)? What is released upon cellular activation? Finally, what is the physiological role of nonopioid fragments derived from these precursors? Numerous studies on dynorphin A 1-17 suggest the presence of a nonopioid action, which often counteracts classical opiate-like effects (206,207). Furthermore, we are beginning to accumulate evidence that opioid systems may liberate a different mix of products depending on their recent regulatory history, as different processing steps become rate-limiting (93,208). It is therefore conceivable that following chronic administration of opiate drugs, the endogenous opioid systems are left with altered biosynthetic capacity as revealed by changes in mRNA. In addition, they may have altered processing patterns and therefore altered mixtures of releasable products (opioid and nonopioid), which would transmit a different message to the receiving neuron. This change in releasable products, coupled with receptors that have been modified to render them less efficacious, would result in dramatically changed opioid unit. How extensive are these changes? How synchronized? How reversible? We need to describe this altered picture at a cellular level so we can begin to understand the long-term behavioral changes observed following acute and repeated administration of opiates. It should be noted that such regulatory studies, though of potential value to the understanding of tolerance, physical dependence, and negative reinforcement, offer little toward the understanding of positive reinforcement. Positive reinforcement is an acute phenomenon, occurring immediately on activation of the proper receptor sites. Regulatory changes, on the other hand, take place over a considerably longer time course. It is therefore a certainty that the acutely reinforcing actions of drugs will fail to be reflected in changes in messenger RNA, peptide processing, or receptor sensitivity. Instead, it is the postreceptor events within the neuron, including second-messenger events and action potential generation or inhibition that will be most important to the understanding of the acute actions of self-administered drugs.

Neuronal Circuits

Current View of the Limbic-Motor Reinforcement Circuit

Our examination of the brain sites involved in the positive reinforcing actions of psychomotor stimulants and opioids, and the efferents and afferents of these structures, has revealed some very interesting and important clues about the neuroanatomy of self-administration. The sites at which opioids have well-documented positive reinforcing actions are the NACC, the LH, and the VTA. Sites important for the positive reinforcing actions of psychomotor stimulants include the NACC and the MPC. The first point that becomes apparent from examination of the neuroanatomy of these sites is that they are not individual, isolated brain sites but are intimately related parts of a circuit. Ventral tegmental area neurons send ascending projections to both the NACC and the MPC, providing the dopamine input to these frontal regions. Neurons of the MPC project back to the VTA and to the NACC. The NACC projects to the LH and the VTA. The VTA, in addition, receives input from the LH. This arrangement provides for a circuit loop in which each of these brain sites communicates monosynaptically with other sites in the loop. The importance of this circuit in positive reinforcement is demonstrated by the fact that each of the nuclei in the circuit supports high rates of self-stimulation behavior in addition to being involved in the reinforcing actions of self-administered drugs. Moreover, each of these sites has been studied for involvement in natural reinforcers, such as food and water intake, and other approach behaviors. This evidence has prompted us to refer to the circuit as the "limbic-motor reinforcement circuit." Although most researcher in the field have recognized the different sites involved in the positive reinfocing actions of opioids and psychomotor stimulants, the sites have been viewed as somewhat independent reinforcement sites. The recognition that these sites are intimately interconnected provides a new vantage point from which to study the neuroanatomy of positive reinforcement and self-administration. For example, what effects will lesions at one site have on reinforcement at another site? Might these multiple sites be involved in redundancy of brain function? What happens to the reinforcing actions of drugs and other positive reinforcers when multiple sites are lesioned?

Examination of the neuroanatomy of the limbic-motor reinforcement circuit has revealed a very interesting and perhaps important convergence at the level of the NACC. As discussed above, while dopamine terminals are distributed throughout the NACC and the dorsal striatum, there is a particularly dense localization in the medial aspect of the NACC. This distribution overlaps the hippocampal input to NACC, as well as very high concentrations of all three opioid receptor types. Outputs of the medial NACC project to the ventral pallidum, the LH and the VTA, as well as other limbic-related brain sites. It therefore appears that opioid receptors and dopamine terminals in the medial NACC are in an excellent position to modulate limbic input to the NACC and motor and limbic output from the NACC. This convergence prompts us to speculate that the NACC may be compartmentalized, with the different subdivisions concerned with different aspects of physiological processes underlying reinforcement. Opioids appear to be associated with the medial subdivision of this nucleus. It will be of interest to compare the medial NACC to more lateral aspects of this nucleus for the reinforcing actions of opioids and psychomotor stimulants. Further analysis of this compartmentalization by selective lesions of the medial versus the lateral NACC or by microinjection of opioids or stimulants into these distinct regions may allow clearer definition of the role of the NACC in emotional and motor aspects of reinforcement.

Future Anatomical Directions

The proposed existence of a positive reinforcement circuit important in drug self-administration should naturally lead us to attempt a better biological integration of its elements. From this perspective we can more fully examine the neurotransmitters and brain sites involved in positive reinforcement and perhaps identify other neurotransmitters that might play a role. For example, neurotensin and neurotensin receptors are found in high concentrations in the VTA. Can this peptide affect reinforcement at the level of the VTA? In fact, a recent study has found that neurotensin is reinforcing when injected into this brain region (209). With this strategy in mind, one can study receptor maps for various neurotransmitters within the limbic-motor reinforcement circuit and speculate as to which receptors might be in a position to modulate or produce reinforcement. Because a number of neurotransmitters and neurotransmitter receptors are found within this circuit, we believe that other substances will undoubtedly be revealed either to be reinforcing or powerful in modifying the reinforcing actions of self-administered drugs.

Additionally, recognition of the limbic-motor reinforcement circuit helps in the identification of afferents and efferents that might be important to the positive reinforcing actions of drugs. The input to the circuit from hippocampus and amygdala are of strong interest, inasmuch as these are classically defined ''limbic'' brain sites, presumably involved in motivation and emotion. Manipulation of these inputs, as well as others, will help to determine the role of afferent activity to the reinforcing actions of drugs. Examination of the outputs of the limbic-motor reinforcement circuit will be of particular interest to researchers in the field. Although opioids and psychomotor stimulants are both reinforcing at the level of the NACC, it is currently unknown whether these substances activate a common output from the NACC or merely closely associated output pathways.

Although many of the questions raised above can be answered by the use of classical techniques, we feel that the emerging technologies will be most useful in elucidating the detailed anatomy of the brain and of the limbic-motor circuit. As the field currently stands, one can easily localize neurotransmitter terminals and the cells producing these transmitters by the use of immunocytochemical and *in situ* hybridization techniques. In the case of receptors, the macromolecules themselves can easily be localized by autoradiography, but we do not yet have the ability to identify the receptor-producing cells. This ability is critical, since the receptor-producing cells are those neurons receiving the neurochemical message, whether it is synaptic release of a neurotransmitter or exogenous administration of a drug. These neurons are therefore **the** translators for the reinforcing message; they are the units that recognize the message, process it, and communicate it to the next neuron in the chain, eventually leading to the physiological impact of the reinforcing stimulus. Therefore, the receptor-producing cells can be viewed as the critical step in reinforcement; their elimination should eliminate the reinforcing actions of the drug in question.

The tools needed to identify the receptor-producing neurons are currently being worked out. One important approach involves cloning the mRNA coding for the opioid receptor of interest in order to localize the receptive neuron by *in situ* hybridization or combined *in situ* hybridization and tract tracing (Figure 2.16). Similarly invaluable for study of the microanatomy of the limbic-motor reinforcement circuit will be the development of selective antibodies to the various receptors. As with the *in situ* analysis, the antibodies may be used in combination with tract-tracing techniques in order to identify receptor-producing neurons. In addition, antibodies produced against a particular receptor when conjugated with lectin-derived neurotoxins or cytotoxic immunoglobins, or both, may allow one to selectively lesion only those neurons that produce the receptor. *In vivo* injection of antibody, followed by binding and subsequent immune- or toxin-mediated lesions may prove to be an

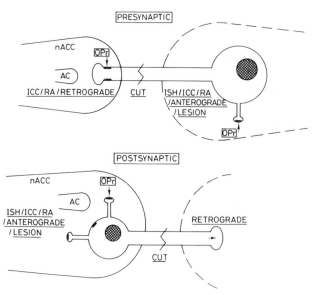

FIGURE 2.16. The two logical possibilities for opiate receptor-producing cells as related to the nucleus accumbens (nACC). Regardless of whether the receptors are *presynaptic* or *postsynaptic*, their cells of origin can be located by immunocytochemistry (ICC), retrograde tract tracing (Retrograde), *in situ* hybridization (ISH), anterograde tract tracing, lesioning of cells, and cutting of axons (CUT). The receptor-rich terminals can be localized by receptor autoradiography (RA). In either case, the opiate receptor–producing structures with inputs to, or receiving outputs from, the nACC can then be studied for their role in reinforcement. This type of high-resolution biochemical anatomy can equally well be applied to other receptor systems, the study of stimulants, and the study of tolerance and dependence.

invaluable tool for identification and disruption of the circuitry of drug action.

Using similar approaches, it is hoped that the elements of the negative reinforcement circuits can be elucidated—in particular, the role of endogenous opioids in this context. It is certain that the positive and negative reinforcement circuits will prove to be closely linked, to have common elements, and to display an integrated output that governs the organism's motivational state and learning patterns.

Integration of Cell Biology and Anatomy

The suggested strategies at both cellular and anatomical levels could generate a veritable deluge of information without yielding a cohesive picture of the biology of drug-seeking behavior. It is therefore critical to keep in mind the key questions in framing any of these studies. What are the *dynamic neurochemical and neurophysiological changes within these circuits* that lead to either the establishment or the maintenance of drug-seeking behavior? In other words, we need to carry out neuronal regulation studies within an anatomical framework. This approach is now rendered particularly feasible by techniques such as quantitative *in situ* hybridization and receptor autoradiography (Figure 2.16). Such tools can also be supplemented with electrophysiological methods and with emerging techniques to quantitate local release of neurotransmitters. As these approaches can be technically demanding, it will be crucial to focus on key anatomical elements—for example, those elements of the circuits that can be seen as the final integrators of their neuronal activity. Thus, in our example of positive reinforcement, we would examine the effect of drugs on the dynamics of NACC output at a very cellular level using the above-mentioned tools, thereby providing a starting point and allowing later incorporation of studies on the dynamics of the input into this nucleus. It is hoped that such strategies could lead us from the cellular and structural level back to the functional level with an understanding of the modification in the overall "tone" of the positive reinforcement or negative reinforcement systems that drive drug-seeking behavior.

Individual Differences

Implicit in all discussions of self-administration of drugs is the question of individual differences. What predisposes some individuals to such behavior and spares others? Discussions of biology versus environment have resulted in little insight. Presupposing a role for each, we can begin to address the question of biology. Are there genetic differences between addiction-prone individuals and their counterparts? The obvious answer is yes since all biology is genetically coded. But does that mean an "addiction gene" in the same way that one hopes to isolate specific genes coding for diseases such as Huntington's disease or even manic-depressive illness? Or should we construe drug seeking as a learned behavior, with genetic predisposition, but no direct linkage to a particular single gene?

While one can reasonably argue either case, it is impossible to settle the question *a priori*. However, it is possible to consider how individual differences in brain organization would lead to varying tendencies to seek and maintain self-administration of certain drugs. The question of variation, which lies at the center of human genetics, has been ill addressed by the brain sciences. This shortcoming reflects our limited understanding of the determinants of the "norm," a knowledge necessary for us to explore the causes of variance. We therefore believe that the strategies outlined above for studying the dynamics of positive and negative reinforcement circuits and their response to reinforcing drugs will provide a cornerstone for addressing the question of individual differences. Can we find individual animals, or better yet inbred strains, with differing propensities towards self-administration? Can we dissociate opiate from psychomotor stimulant self-administration? Do these animals differ in the "tone" of their positive reinforcement circuits, or in the relative "tone" of positive and negative reinforcement circuits? Can these differences be traced back to differences in relative receptor number or affinities? To neuronal organization? To developmental events?

There is no guarantee that such studies will lead us to the answers in the human situation. They will merely point to certain possibilities and will force us to seek answers to the question of variance as well as to understanding the mean.

Conclusions

In this review we have attempted to describe the biochemical and anatomical substrates of drug-seeking behavior with particular emphasis on opiate drugs and endogenous opioid systems. In addition we have attempted to describe future research strategies that could help us achieve a better understanding of this unusual behavior.

Avram Goldstein, in an early review on opioid peptides and receptors in the brain commented "it seemed unlikely, a priori, that such highly stereospecific receptors should have been developed by nature to interact with alkaloids from the opium poppy" (210). To paraphrase Dr. Goldstein, it seems highly unlikely that systems in the brain should have been developed by nature for the self-administration of exogenous substances. Nature developed brain systems for reinforcement function, not for self-administration of drugs. The fact that some individuals choose to activate these systems chemically, through drug administration, reflects the power that these systems have on behavior. It also forces us to face certain basic questions regarding the way brain biology can control behavior and the way that behavior, in turn, can alter brain biology.

Acknowledgments. We would like to thank Carrie Sercel for smiles and secretarial assistance above and beyond the call of duty, and Kathy Koppelo, Sharon Burke, and Giulio Baldrighi for assistance with the figures. Alfred Mansour provided helpful discussions about the opioid receptors, as well as Figure 2.15. This work was supported by NIDA National Research Service Award DA05336 (K.A.T.), NIA National Research Service Award AG000123 (J.P.H.), MH422251 (H.A., S.W.), NIDA DA02265 (H.A., S.W.), and Theophile Raphael Research Fund (H.A.).

References

1. Edwards G, Arif A, Hodgson R (1981). Nomenclature and classification of drug- and alcohol-related problems: A WHO memorandum. *Bull. WHO* 59:225–242.
2. Skinner BF (1938). *The Behavior of Organisms: An Experimental Analysis.* Appleton, New York.
3. Jaffe JH (1980). Drug addiction and drug abuse. In AG Gilman, LS Goodman, A Gilman, eds. *The Pharmacological Basis of Therapeutics.* Macmillan, New York, pp 535–584.
4. Olds J, Milner P (1954). Positive reinforcement produced by electrical stimulation of septal area and other regions. *J Comp Physiol Psychol* 47:419–427.
5. Olds J (1977). *Drives and Reinforcements: Behavioral Studies of Hypothalamic Functions.* Raven Press, New York.
6. Stein L (1978). Reward transmitters: Catecholamines and opioid peptides. In MA Lipton, A DiMascio, KF Killam, eds. *Psychopharmacology: A Generation of Progress.* Raven Press, New York, pp 569–581.
7. Ebin D (1961). *The Drug Experience.* Orion Press, New York.
8. Bozarth MA (1987). *Methods of Assessing the Reinforcing Properties of Abused Drugs.* Springer-Verlag, New York.
9. Himmelsbach CK (1943). With reference to physical dependence. *Fed Proc* 2:201–203.
10. Lindsmith AR (1947). *Opiate Addiction.* Principia Press, Bloomington, IN.
11. Martin WR (1968). A homeostatic and redundancy theory of tolerance and dependence to narcotic analgesics. *Res Publ Assoc Res Nerv Ment Dis* 46:206–225.
12. Deneau G, Yanagita T, Seever MH (1969). Self-administration of psychoactive substances by the monkey: A measure of psychological dependence. *Psychopharmacology (Berlin)* 16:30–48.
13. Johanson CE, Balster RL, Bonese K (1976). Self-administration of psychomotor stimulant drugs: The effects of unlimited access. *Pharmacol Biochem Behav* 4:45–51.
14. Jones BE, Prada JA (1977). Drug-seeking behavior in the dog: Lack of effect of prior passive dependence on morphine. *Drug Alc Depend.* 2:287–294.
15. Koob GF (1987). Neural substrates of opioid tolerance and dependence. In *Problems of Drug Dependence.* Research Monograph 76. National Institute on Drug Abuse Research, Rockville, MD, pp 46–52.

16. Zinberg NE, Harding WM, Stelmack SM, Marblestone RA (1978). Patterns of heroin use. *Ann NY Acad Sci* 311:10–24.
17. Harding WM, Zinberg NE (1983). Occasional opiate use. *Adv Substance Abuse* 3:27–61.
18. Gilman AG, Goodman LS, Gilman A, eds. (1980). *The Pharmacological Basis of Therapeutics,* Macmillan, New York.
19. Goldberg SR, Hoffmeister, F, Schichting U, Wuttke W (1971). Aversive properties of nalorphine and naloxone in morphine dependent rhesus monkeys. *J Pharmacol Exp Ther* 179:268.
20. Dackis CA, Gold MS (1985). New concepts in cocaine addiction: The dopamine depletion hypothesis. *Neurosci Behav Rev* 9:469–477.
21. O'Brien CP, Ehrman RN, Ternes JW (1986). Classical conditioning in human opioid dependence. In SR Goldberg, IP Stolerman, eds. *Behavioral Analysis of Drug Dependence.* Academic Press, Orlando, FL, pp 329–356.
22. Ryberg U (1986). Alcohol withdrawal and opiate withdrawal—similarities and differences. *Acta Psychiat Scand* 73(Suppl):61–73.
23. Wei E, Loh HH, Way EL (1973). Brain sites of precipitated abstinence in morphine-dependent rats. *J Pharmacol Exp Ther* 185:108–115.
24. Wei E, Sigel SSR, Loh HH, Way EL (1975). Central sites of naloxone-precipitated shaking in the anesthetized, morphine-dependent rat. *J Pharmacol Exp Ther* 195:480–487.
25. Bechara A, van der Kooy D (1987). Separation of morphine's incentive motivational from its escape from withdrawal properties. *Soc Neurosci Abstr* 13:1547.
26. Kuczenski R (1983). Biochemical actions of amphetamine and other stimulants. In I Creese, ed. *Stimulants: Neurochemical, Behavioral, and Clinical Perspectives,* Raven Press, New York, pp 31–61.
27. Greenshaw AJ (1984). β-Phenylethylamine and reinforcement. *Progr Neuropsychopharmacol* 8:615–620.
28. Wise RA (1982). Neuroleptics and operant behavior: The anhedonia hypothesis. *Behav Brain Sci* 5:39–87.
29. Fibiger HG, Phillips AG (1986). Reward, motivation, cognition: Psychobiology of mesotelencephalic dopamine systems. In VB Mountcastle, FE Bloom, SR Geiger, eds. *Handbook of Physiology: The Nervous System IV.* American Physiological Society, Bethesda, MD, pp 647–675.
30. Davis WM, Smith SG (1975). Effect of haloperidol on (+)-amphetamine self-administration. *J Pharm Pharmac* 27:540–542.
31. De Wit H, Wise RA (1977). Blockade of cocaine reinforcement in rats with the dopamine receptor blocker pimozide, but not with the noradrenergic blockers phentolamine or phenoxybenzamine. *Can J Psychol* 31:195–203.
32. Risner ME, Jones BE (1976). Role of noradrenergic and dopaminergic processes in amphetamine self-administration. *Pharmac Biochem Behav* 5:477–482.
33. Yokel RA, Wise RA (1975). Increased lever pressing for amphetamine after pimozide in rats: Implications for a dopamine theory of reward. *Science* 187:547–549.
34. Yokel RA, Wise RA (1976). Attenuation of intravenous amphetamine reinforcement by central dopamine blockade in rats. *Psychopharmacology (Berlin)* 48:311–318.

35. Spyraki C, Fibiger HC, Phillips AG (1982). Dopaminergic substrates of amphetamine-induced place preference conditioning. *Brain Res* 253:185–193.
36. Mackey WB, van der Kooy D (1985). Neuroleptics block the positive reinforcing effects of amphetamine but not of morphine as measured by place conditioning. *Pharmacol Biochem Behav* 22:101–105.
37. Mithani S, Martin-Iverson MT, Phillips AG, Fibiger HC (1986). The effects of haloperidol on amphetamine- and methylphenidate-induced conditioned place preferences and locomotor activity. *Psychopharmacology (Berlin)* 90:247–252.
38. Morency MA, Beninger RJ (1986). Dopaminergic substrates of cocaine-induced place conditioning. *Brain Res* 399:33–41.
39. Jonsson L, Anggard E, Gunne L (1971). Blockade of intravenous amphetamine euphoria in man. *Clin Pharmacol Ther* 12:889–896.
40. Lyness WH, Friedle NM, Moore KE (1979). Destruction of dopaminergic nerve terminals in nucleus accumbens: Effect on D-amphetamine self-administration. *Pharmacol Biochem Behav* 11:553–556.
41. Roberts DCS, Koob GF, Klonoff P, Fibiger HC (1980). Extinction and recovery of cocaine self-administration following 6-hydroxydopamine lesions of the nucleus accumbens. *Pharmacol Biochem Behav* 12:781–787.
42. Pettit HO, Ettenberg A, Bloom FE, Koob GF (1984). Destruction of dopamine in the nucleus accumbens selectively attenuates cocaine but not heroin self-administration in rats. *Psychopharmacology (Berlin)* 84:167–173.
43. Monaco AP, Hernandez L, Hoebel BG (1981). Nucleus accumbens: Site of amphetamine self-injection: Comparison with the lateral ventricle. In RB Chronister, J DeFrance, eds. *The Neurobiology of the Nucleus Accumbens* Haer Institute, Brunswick, ME, pp 338–342.
44. Hoebel BG, Monaco AP, Hernandez L, Aulisi EF, Stanley BG, Lenard L (1983). Self-injection of amphetamine directly into the brain. *Psychopharmacology (Berlin)* 81:158–163.
45. Carr GD, White NM (1983). Conditioned place preference from intra-accumbens but not intra-caudate amphetamine injections. *Life Sci* 33:2551–2557.
46. Carr GD, White NM (1986). Anatomical disassociation of amphetamine's rewarding and aversive effects: An intracranial microinjection study. *Psychopharmacology (Berlin)* 89:340–346.
47. Taylor JR, Robbins TW (1984). Enhanced behavioural control by conditioned reinforcers following microinjections of d-amphetamine into the nucleus accumbens. *Psychopharmacology (Berlin)* 84:405–412.
48. Aulisi EF, Hoebel BG (1983). Rewarding effects of amphetamine and cocaine in the nucleus accumbens and block by flupenthixol. *Soc Neurosci Abstr* 9:121.
49. Goeders NE, Smith JE (1983). Cortical dopaminergic involvement in cocaine reinforcement. *Science* 221:773–775.
50. Goeders NE, Dworkin SI, Smith JE (1986). Neuropharmacological assessment of cocaine self-administration into the medial prefrontal cortex. *Pharmacol Biochem Behav* 24:1429–1440.
51. Goeders NE, Smith JE (1986). Reinforcing properties of cocaine in the medial prefrontal cortex: Primary action on presynaptic dopaminergic terminals. *Pharmacol Biochem Behav* 25:191–199.

52. Guerin GF, Goeders NE, Dworkin SI, Smith JE (1984). Intracranial self-administration of dopamine into the nucleus accumbens. *Soc Neurosci Abstr* 10:1072.
53. Woolverton WL (1986). Effects of D_1 and a D_2 dopamine antagonist on the self-administration of cocaine and piribedil by rhesus monkeys. *Pharmacol Biochem Behav* 24:531–535.
54. Gallistel CR, Davis AJ (1983). Affinity for the dopamine D_2 receptor predicts neuroleptic potency in blocking the reinforcing effect of MFB stimulation. *Pharmacol Biochem Behav* 19:867–872.
55. Walters JR, Bergstrom DA, Carlson JH, Chase TN, Braun AR (1987). D_1 dopamine receptor activation required for postsynaptic expression of D_2 agonist effects. *Science* 236:719–722.
56. Creese I, Iversen SD (1975). The pharmacological and anatomical substrates of the amphetamine response in rat. *Brain Res* 83:419–436.
57. Kelly PH, Seviour PW, Iversen SD (1975). Amphetamine and apomorphine responses in the rat following 6-OHDA lesions of the nucleus accumbens septi and corpus striatum. *Brain Res* 94:507–522.
58. Holtzman SG (1976). Comparison of the effects of morphine, pentazocine, cyclazocine and amphetamine on intracranial self-stimulation in the rat. *Psychopharmacologia (Berlin)* 46:223–227.
59. Esposito RU, Perry W, Kornetsky C (1980). Effects of D-amphetamine and naloxone on brain stimulation reward. *Psychopharmacology* 69:187–191.
60. Trujillo KA, Belluzzi JD, Stein L (1983). Endorphin-catecholamine interactions in nucleus accumbens self-stimulation. *Soc Neurosci Abstr* 9:277.
61. Trujillo KA, Belluzzi JD, Tabrizi PR, Stein L (1985). Naloxone blockade of amphetamine reward in place preference conditioning. *Soc Neurosci Abstr* 11:1173.
62. Bain GT, Kornetsky C (1986). Naloxone attenuation of the effect of cocaine on rewarding brain stimulation. *Life Sci* 40:1119–1125.
63. Carroll ME, Lac ST, Walker MJ, Kragh R, Newman T (1986). Effects of naltrexone on intravenous cocaine self-administration in rats during food satiation and deprivation. *J Pharmacol Exp Ther* 238:1–7.
64. Umemoto M, Olds ME (1981). Presynaptic alpha-adrenergic mediation of self-stimulation in locus coeruleus in rats treated neonatally with 6-hydroxydopamine. *Brain Res* 219:107–119.
65. Cytawa J, Jurkowlaniec E, Bialowas J (1980). Positive reinforcement produced by noradrenergic stimulation of the hypothalamus in rats. *Physiol Behav* 25:615–619.
66. Shearman GT, Hynes M, Lal H (1981). Self-administration of clonidine by the rat. In H Lal, S Fielding, eds. *Psychopharmacology of Clonidine*. Alan R Liss, New York, pp 259–276.
67. Hughes J, Smith TW, Kosterlitz HW, Fothergill LA, Morgan BA, Morris HR (1975). Identification of two related pentapeptides from the brain with potent opiate agonist activity. *Nature (London)* 258:577–579.
68. Noda M, Teranishi Y, Takahashi H, Toyosato M, Notake M, Nakanishi S, Numa S (1982). Isolation and structural organization of the human pre-proenkephalin gene. *Nature (London)* 297:431–434.
69. Comb J, Herbert E, Crea R (1982). Partial characterization of the mRNA that codes for enkephalins in bovine adrenal medulla and human pheochromocytoma. *Proc Natl Acad Sci USA* 79:360–364.

70. Kimura S, Lewis RV, Stern AS, Rossier J, Stein S, Udenfriend S (1980). Probable precursors of (Leu) enkephalin and (Met) enkephalin in adrenal medulla: Peptides of 3–5 kilodaltons. *Proc Natl Acad Sci USA* 77:1681–1685.
71. Li CH, Chung D (1976). Isolation and structure of an untriakontapeptide with opiate activity from camel pituitary glands. *Proc Natl Acad Sci USA* 73:1145–1148.
72. Nakanishi S, Inoue A, Kita T, Nakamura M, Chang ACY, Cohen SN, Numa S (1979). Nucleotide sequence of cloned cDNA for bovine corticotropin-beta-lipotropin precursor. *Nature (London)* 278:423–427.
73. Goldstein A, Tachibana S, Lowney LI, Hunkapiller M, Hood L (1979). Dynorphin-(1-13), an extraordinarily potent opioid peptide. *Proc Natl Acad Sci USA* 76:6666–6670.
74. Kakidani H, Furutani Y, Takehashi H, Noda M, Morimoto Y, Hirone T, Asai M, Inayama S, Nakanishi S, Numa S (1982). Cloning and sequence analysis of cDNA for porcine beta-neo-endorphin, dynorphin precursor. *Nature (London)* 298:245–249.
75. Day R, Akil H (1986). Bridge peptide is a cleavage product of pro-dynorphin processing in the rat anterior pituitary. In *Advances in Endogenous and Exogenous Opioid Peptides (INRC Proceedings)*. NIDA Research Monograph 75. US Department of Health and Human Services, Washington, DC, pp 244–276.
76. Richter K, Egger R, Kreil G (1987). D-Alanine in the frog skin peptide dermorphin is derived from L-alanine in the precursor. *Science* 238:200–202.
77. Donnerer J, Oka K, Brossi A, Rice KC, Spector S (1986). Presence and formation of codeine and morphine in the rat. *Proc Natl Acad Sci USA* 83:4566–4567.
78. Goldstein A, Barrett RW, James IF, Lowney LI, Weitz CJ, Knipmeyer LL, Rapoport H (1985). Morphine and other opiates from beef brain and adrenal. *Proc Natl Acad Sci USA* 82:5203–5207.
79. Weitz CJ, Faull KF, Goldstein A (1988). Synthesis of the skeleton of the morphine molecule by mammalian liver. *Nature (London)* 330:674–677.
80. Martin WR (1984). Pharmacology of opioids. *Pharmacol Rev* 35:283–323.
81. Wood PL (1982). Multiple opiate receptors: Support for unique mu, delta and kappa sites. *Neuropharmacology* 24:487–497.
82. Schulz R, Wuster M, Herz A (1981). Pharmacological characterization of the ε-opiate receptor. *J Pharmacol Exp Ther* 216:604–606.
83. Werz MA, Macdonald RL (1983). Opioid peptides selective for mu and delta receptors reduce calcium dependent action potentials by increasing potassium conductance. *Neurosci Lett* 42:173–178.
84. Werz MA, Macdonald RL (1983). Opioid peptides with differential affinity for mu and delta receptors decrease sensory neuron calcium-dependent action potentials. *J Pharmacol Exp Ther* 227:394–402.
85. North RA (1986). Membrane conductances and opioid receptor subtypes. In RM Brown, DH Clouet, DP Friedman, eds. *Opiate Receptor Subtypes and Brain Function*. NIDA Research Monograph 71. US Department of Health and Human Services, Washington, DC, pp 81–88.
86. North RA, Williams JT, Surprenant A, Christie MJ (1987). Mu and Delta receptors belong to a family of receptors that are coupled to potassium channels. *Proc Natl Acad Sci USA* 84:5487–5491.
87. Werz MA, MacDonald RL (1984). Dynorphin reduces calcium-dependent

action potential duration by decreasing voltage-dependent calcium conductance. *Neurosci Lett* 46:185–190.

88. Werz MA, Macdonald RL (1984). Dynorphin reduces voltage-dependent calcium conductance of mouse dorsal root ganglion neurons. *Neuropeptides* 5:253–256.

89. Werz MA, Macdonald RL (1985). Dynorphin and neo-endorphin peptides decrease dorsal root ganglion neuron calcium-dependent action potential duration. *J Pharmacol Exp Ther* 234:49–56.

90. Cherubini E, North RA (1985). Mu and kappa opioids inhibit transmitter release by different mechanisms. *Proc Natl Acad Sci USA* 82:1860–1863.

91. Wollemann M (1981). Endogenous opioids and cyclic AMP. *Progr Neurobiol* 16:145–154.

92. Childers SR, Nijssen P, Nadeau P, Buckhanna P, Le PV, Harris J (1986). Opiate-inhibited adenylate cyclase in mammalian brain membranes. In RM Brown, DH Clouet, DP Friedman, eds. *Opiate Receptor Subtypes and Brain Function*. NIDA Research Monograph 71. US Department of Health and Human Services, Washington, DC, pp 65–80.

93. Watson SJ, Akil H, Young E (1987). Hypothalamic-pituitary-adrenal axis peptides in affective disease: Focus on the ACTH/β-endorphin system. In CB Nemeroff, PF Loosen eds. *Handbook of Clinical Psychoneuroendocrinology*. Guilford, New York, pp 384–396.

94. Gramsch C, Kleber G, Volker H, Pasi A, Mehraein P, Herz A (1980). Pro-opiocortin fragments in human and rat brain: Beta-endorphin and alpha-MSH are predominant peptides. *Brain Res* 192:109–119.

95. Dores RM, Jain M, Akil H (1986). Characterization of the forms of β-endorphin and α-MSh in the caual medulla of the rat and guinea pig. *Brain Res* 377:251–260.

96. Seizinger BR, Grimm C, Hollt V, Herz A (1984). Evidence for a selective processing of proenkephalin B into different opioid peptide forms in particular regions of rat brain and pituitary. *J Neurochem* 42:447–457.

97. Trujillo KA, Day R, Akil H (1987). Increases in striatonigral dynorphins following repeated amphetamine injections. *Soc Neurosci Abstr* 13:637.

98. Weeks JR, Collins RJ (1976). Changes in morphine self-administration in rats induced by prostaglandin E and naloxone. *Prostaglandins* 12:11–19.

99. Ettenberg A, Pettit HO, Bloom FE, Koob GF (1982). Heroin and cocaine intravenous self-administration in rats: Mediation by separate neural systems. *Psychopharmacology* 78:204–209.

100. Koob GF, Pettit HO, Ettenberg A, Bloom FE (1984). Effects of opiate antagonists and their quaternary derivatives on heroin self-administration in the rat. *J Pharmacol Exp Ther* 229:481–485.

101. Vaccarino FJ, Pettit HO, Bloom FE, Koob GF (1985). Effects of intracerebroventricular administration of methyl naloxonium chloride on heroin self-administration in the rat. *Pharmacol Biochem Behav* 23:495–498.

102. Bozarth MA, Wise RA (1981). Heroin reward is dependent on a dopaminergic substrate. *Life Sci* 29:1881–1886.

103. Phillips AG, LePiane FG (1982). Reward produced by microinjection of (D-Ala^2), Met^5-enkephalinamide into the ventral tegmental area. *Behav Brain Res* 5:225–229.

104. Phillips AG, LePiane FG, Fibiger HC (1983). Dopaminergic mediation of

reward produced by direct injection of enkephalin into the ventral tegmental area of the rat. *Life Sci* 33:2505–2511.
105. Spyraki C, Fibiger HC, Phillips AG (1983). Attenuation of heroin reward in rats by disruption of the mesolimbic dopamine system. *Psychopharmacology* 79:278–283.
106. Bozarth MA, Wise RA (1986). Involvement of the ventral tegmental dopamine system in opioid and psychomotor stimulant reinforcement. In LH Harris, ed. *Problems of Drug Dependence.* NIDA Research Monograph 67. US Department of Health and Human Services, Washington, DC, pp 190–196.
107. Bozarth MA (1986). Neural basis of psychomotor stimulant and opiate reward: Evidence suggesting the involvement of a common dopaminergic system.*Behav Brain Res* 22:107–116.
108. Koob GF (in press). Separate neurochemical substrates for cocaine and heroin reinforcement. In ML Commons, ed. *Quantitative Analyses of Behavior: Biological Determinants of Behavior, vol. 7.* Erlbaum, Hillsdale, NJ.
109. Schwartz AS, Marchok PL (1974). Depression of morphine-seeking behavior by dopamine inhibition. *Nature (London)* 248:257–258.
110. Broekkamp CLE, Phillips AG, Cools AR (1979). Facilitation of self-stimulation behavior following intracranial microinjections of opioids into the ventral tegmental area. *Pharmacol Biochem Behav* 11:289–295.
111. Stinus L, Koob GF, Ling N, Bloom FE, Le Moal M (1980). Locomotor activation induced by infusion of endorphins into the ventral tegmental area: Evidence for opiate-dopamine interactions. *Proc Natl Acad Sci USA* 77:2323–2327.
112. Gysling K, Wang RY (1983). Morphine-induced activation of A10 dopamine neurons in the rat. *Brain Res* 277:119–127.
113. Matthews RT, German DC (1984). Electrophysiologial evidence for excitation of rat ventral tegmental area dopaminergic neurons by morphine. *Neuroscience* 11:617–625.
114. Di Chiara G, Imperato A (1986). Preferential stimulation of dopamine release in the nucleus accumbens by opiates, alcohol, and barbiturates: Studies with transcerebral dialysis in freely moving rats. *Ann NY Acad Sci* 473:367–381.
115. Bozarth MA, Wise RA (1981). Intracranial self-administration of morphine into the ventral tegmental area in rats. *Life Sci* 28:551–555.
116. Olds ME, Williams KN (1980). Self-administration of d-Ala-Met-Enkephalinamide at hypothalamic self-stimulation sites. *Brain Res* 194:155–170.
117. Cazala P, Darrac C, Saint-Marc M (1987). Self-administration of morphine into the lateral hypothalamus in the mouse. *Brain Res* 416:283–288.
118. Olds ME (1982). Reinforcing effects of morphine in the nucleus accumbens. *Brain Res* 237:429–440.
119. Goeders NE, Lane JD, Smith JE (1984). Self-administration of methionine enkephalin into the nucleus accumbens. *Pharmacol Biochem Behav* 20, 451–455.
120. van der Kooy D, Mucha RF, O'Shaughnessy M, Buceneiks P (1982). Reinforcing effects of brain microinjections of morphine revealed by conditioned place preferences. *Brain Res* 243:107–117.

121. Romer D, Hill RC, Maurer R (1982). Receptor interactions and reinforcing capacities of different opioids. In S Saito, T Yanagita ,eds. *Learning and Memory Drugs as Reinforcers.* Excerpta Medica, Amsterdam, pp 286–293.

122. Mucha RF, Herz A (1985). Motivational properties of kappa and mu opioid receptor agonists studied with place and taste preference conditioning. *Psychopharmacology* 86:274–280.

123. Pfeiffer A, Brantl V, Herz A, Emrich HM (1986). Psychotomimesis mediated by kappa opiate receptors. *Science* 233:774–776.

124. Jenck F, Gratton A, Wise RA (1987). Opioid receptor subtypes associated with ventral tegmental facilitation of lateral hypothalamic brain stimulation reward. *Brain Res* 423, 34–38.

125. Shippenberg TS, Bals-Kubik R, Herz A (1987). Motivational properties of opioids: Evidence that an activation of δ-receptors mediates reinforcement processes. *Brain Res* 436:234–239.

126. Pert A, Sivit C (1977). Neuroanatomical focus for morphine and enkephalin-induced hypermotility. *Nature (London)* 265:645–647.

127. Pert A, DeWald A, Liao H, Sivit C (1979). Effects of opiates and opioid peptides on motor behaviors: Sites and mechanisms of action. In E Usdin, NS Kline, WM Bunney, eds. *Endorphins in Mental Health Research.* Macmillan, New York, pp 45–61.

128. Kalivas PW, Widerlov E, Stanley D, Breese G, Prange AJ (1983). Enkephalin action on the mesolimbic system: A dopamine-dependent and a dopamine-independent increase in locomotor activity. *J Pharmacol Exp Ther* 227:229–237.

129. Glickman SE, Schiff BB (1967). A biological theory of reinforcement. *Psychol Rev* 74:81–109.

130. Iversen SD (1983). Brain endorphins and reward function: Some thoughts and speculations. In JE Smith, JD Lane, eds. *The Neurobiology of Opiate Reward Processes.* Elsevier, New York, pp 439–468.

131. Swerdlow NR, Vaccarino FJ, Amalric M, Koob GF (1986). The neural substrates for the motor-activating properties of psychostimulants: A review of recent findings. *Pharmacol Biochem Behav* 25:233–248.

132. Trujillo KA, Akil H, Watson SJ (in press). The biological mechanisms of drugs of abuse. In JD Barchas, PA Berger, RD Ciaranello, GR Elliott, eds. *Psychopharmacology: From Theory to Practice,* 2nd ed. Oxford University Press, New York.

133. Wise RA, Bozarth MA (1987). A psychomotor stimulant theory of addiction. *Psychol Rev* 94:469–492.

134. Trujillo KA, Pert A (1980). Differential behavioral effects of Type I and Type II opiate receptor activation in rat brain. *Soc Neurosci Abstr* 6:36.

135. Carr GD, Phillips AG, Fibiger HC (1988). Independence of amphetamine reward from locomotor stimulation demonstrated by conditioned place preference. *Psychopharmacology* 94:221–226.

136. Mogenson GJ, Jones DL, Yim CY (1980). From motivation to action: Functional interface between the limbic system and the motor system. *Progr Neurobiol* 14:69–97.

137. Mogenson GJ (1982). Studies of the nucleus accumbens and its mesolimbic dopaminergic afferents in relation to ingestive behaviors and reward. In BG Hoebel, D Novin, eds. *The Neural Basis of Feeding and Reward.* Haer Institute, Brunswick, ME, pp 275–287.

138. Yim CY, Mogenson GJ (1982). Response of nucleus accumbens neurons to amygdala stimulation and its modification by dopamine. *Brain Res* 239:401–415.
139. Yim CY, Mogenson GJ (1983). Response of ventral pallidal neurons to amygdala stimulation and its modulation by dopamine projections to nucleus accumbens. *J Neurophysiol* 50:148–161.
140. Yim CY, Mogenson GJ (1986). Mesolimbic dopamine projection modulates amygdala-evoked EPSP in nucleus accumbens neurons: An *in vivo* study. *Brain Res* 369:347–352.
141. Fallon JH, Loughlin SE (1987). Monoamine innervation of cerebral cortex and a theory of the role of monoamines in cerebral cortex and basal ganglia. In EG Jones, A Peters, eds. *Cerebral Cortex,* vol. 6. Plenum, New York, pp 41–127.
142. Fallon JH, Loughlin SE (1985). Substantia nigra.In G Paxinos, ed. *The Rat Nervous System: Forebrain and Midbrain.* vol 1. Academic Press, Orlando, FL, pp 353–374.
143. Hokfelt T, Skirboll L, Rehfeld JF, Goldstein M, Markey K, Dann O (1980). A subpopulation of mesencephalic dopamine neurons projecting to limbic areas contains a cholecystokinin-like peptide: Evidence from immunohistochemistry combined with retrograde tracing. *Neuroscience* 5:2093–2124.
144. Seroogy KB, Mehta A, Fallon JH (1987). Neurotensin and cholecystokinin coexistence within neurons of the ventral mesencephalon: Projections to forebrain. *Exp Brain Res* 68:277–289.
145. Hokfelt T, Everitt BJ, Theodorsson-Norheim E, Goldstein M (1984). Occurrence of neurotensinlike immunoreactivity in subpopulations of hypothalamic, mesencephalic, and medullary catecholamine neurons. *J Comp Neurol* 222:543–559.
146. Kalivas PW, Miller JS (1984). Neurotensin neurons in the ventral tegmental area project to the medial nucleus accumbens. *Brain Res* 300:157–160.
147. Chronister RB, Sikes RW, Trow TW, DeFrance JF (1981). The organization of nucleus accumbens. In RB Chronister, JF DeFrance, eds. *The Neurobiology of the Nucleus Accumbens.* Haer Institute, Brunswick, ME, pp 97–146.
148. Groenewegen HJ, Arnolds DEAT, Lopes da Silva FH (1981). Afferent connections of the nucleus accumbens in the cat, with special emphasis on the projections from the hippocampal region: An anatomical and electrophysiological study. In RB Chronister, JF DeFrance, eds. *The Neurobiology of the Nucleus Accumbens.* Haer Institute, Brunswick, ME, pp 41–74.
149. Krayniak PF, Meibach RC, Siegel A (1981). A projection from the entorhinal cortex to the nucleus accumbens in the rat. *Brain Res* 209:427–431.
150. Zaborszky L, Alheid GF, Beinfeld MC, Eiden LE, Heimer L, Palkovits M (1985). Cholecystokinin innervation of the ventral striatum: A morphological and radioimmunological study. *Neuroscience* 14:427–453.
151. Phillipson OT, Griffiths AC (1985). The topographic order of inputs to nucleus accumbens in the rat. *Neuroscience* 16:275–296.
152. Domesick VB (1981). Further observations on the anatomy of nucleus accumbens and caudate putamen in the rat: Similarities and contrasts. In RB Chronister, JF DeFrance, eds. *The Neurobiology of the Nucleus Accumbens.* Haer Institute, Brunswick, ME, pp 7–39.

153. Kelley AE, Domesick VB (1982). The distribution of the projection from the hippocampal formation to the nucleus accumbens in the rat: An anterograde-and retrograde-horseradish peroxidase study. *Neuroscience* 7:2321–2335.
154. Krettek JE, Price JL (1978). Amygdaloid projections to subcortical structures within the basal forebrain and brainstem in the rat and cat. *J Comp Neurol* 178:225–254.
155. Kelley AE, Domesick VB, Nauta WJH (1982). The amygdalostriatal projection in the rat—An anatomical study by anterograde and retrograde tracing methods. *J Neurosci* 7:615–630.
156. Fuller TA, Russchen FT, Price JL (1987). Sources of presumptive glutamergic/aspartergic afferents to the rat ventral striatopallidal region. *J Comp Neurol* 258:317–338.
157. Groenewegen HJ, Russchen FT (1984). Organization of the efferent projections of the nucleus accumbens to pallidal, hypothalamic, and mesencephalic structures: A tracing and immunohistochemical study in the cat. *J Comp Neurol* 223:347–367.
158. Swanson LW, Cowan WM (1975). A note on the connections and development of the nucleus accumbens. *Brain Res* 92:324–330.
159. Powell EW, Leman RB (1976). Connections of the nucleus accumbens. *Brain Res* 105:389–403.
160. Nauta WJH, Smith GP, Faull RLM, Domesick VB (1978). Efferent connections and nigral afferents of the nucleus accumbens septi in the rat. *Neuroscience* 3:385–401.
161. Jones DL, Mogenson GJ (1980). Nucleus accumbens to globus pallidus gaba projection: Electrophysiological and iontophoretic investigations. *Brain Res* 188:93–105.
162. Mogenson GJ, Swanson LW, Wu M (1983). Neural projections from nucleus accumbens to globus pallidus, substantia innominata, and lateral preopticlateral hypothalamic area: An anatomical and electrophysiological investigation in the rat. *J Neurosci* 3:189–202.
163. Walaas I, Fonnum F (1980). Biochemical evidence for gamma-aminobutyrate containing fibres from the nucleus accumbens to the substantia nigra and ventral tegmental area in the rat. *Neuroscience* 5:63–72.
164. Sugimoto T, Mizuno N (1987). Neurotensin in projection neurons of the striatum and nucleus accumbens, with reference to coexistence with enkephalin and GABA: An immunohistochemical study in the cat. *J Comp Neurol* 257:383–395.
165. Oades RD, Halliday GM (1987). Ventral tegmental (A10) system: Neurobiology. 1. Anatomy and connectivity. *Brain Res Bull* 12:117–165.
166. Swanson LW (1982). The projections of the ventral tegmental area and adjacent regions: A combined fluorescent retrograde tracer and immunofluorescence study in the rat. *Brain Res Bull* 9:321–353.
167. Phillipson OT (1979). Afferent projections to the ventral tegmental area of tsai and interfascicular nucleus: A horseradish peroxidase study in the rat. *J Comp Neurol* 187:117–144.
168. Simon H, LeMoal M, Calas A (1979). Efferents and afferents of the ventral tegmental-A10 region studied after local injection of ^{3}H-leucine and horseradish peroxidase. *Brain Res* 178:17–40.
169. Nauta WJH, Domesick VB (1978). Cross-roads of limbic and striatal

circuitry: Hypothalamo-nigral connections. In KE Livingstone, O Hornykie-wicz, eds. *Limbic Mechanisms: The Continuing Evolution of the Limbic System Concept.* Plenum, New York, pp 75–83.

170. Khachaturian H, Lewis ME, Tsou K, Watson SJ (1985). β-Endorphin, α-MSH, ACTH, and related peptides. In A Bjorklund, T Hokfelt, eds. *Handbook of Chemical Neuroanatomy.* pt 1, *GABA and Neuropeptides in the CNS* vol. 4. Elsevier, New York, pp 216–272.

171. Fallon JH, Leslie FM (1986). Distribution of dynorphin and enkephalin peptides in the rat brain. *J Comp Neurol* 249:293–336.

172. Harlan RE, Shivers BD, Romano GJ, Howells RD, Pfaff DW (1987). Localization of preproenkephalin mRNA in the rat brain and spinal cord by *in situ* hybridization. J Comp Neurol 258:159–184.

173. Khachaturian H, Lewis ME, Hollt V, Watson SJ (1983). Telencephalic enkephalinergic systems in the rat brain. *J Neurosci* 3:844–855.

174. Mansour A, Khachaturian H, Lewis ME, Akil H, Watson SJ (1987). Autoradiographic differentiation of mu, delta, and kappa opioid receptors in the rat forebrain and midbrain. *J Neurosci* 7:2445–2464.

175. Mansour A, Khachaturian H, Lewis ME, Akil H, Watson SJ (1988). Anatomy of CNS opioid receptors. *Trends Neurosci* 11:308–314.

176. Fallon JH, Leslie FM, Cone RI (1985). Dynorphin-containing pathways in the substantia nigra and ventral tegmentum: A double labeling study using combined immunofluorescence and retrograde tracing. *Neuropeptides* 5:457–460.

177. Swanson LW, Mogenson GJ (1981). Neural mechanisms for the functional coupling of autonomic, endocrine, and somatomotor responses in adapative behavior. *Brain Res Rev* 3:1–34.

178. Bozarth MA (1987). Neuroanatomical boundaries of the reward-relevant opiate-receptor field in the ventral tegmental area as mapped by the conditioned place preference method in rats. *Brain Res* 414:77–86.

179. Williams JT, North RA (1984). Opioid-receptor interactions on single locus coeruleus neurons. *Molec Pharmacol* 26:489–497.

180. Aghajanian GK (1978). Tolerance of locus coeruleus neurons to morphine and suppression of withdrawal response by clonidine. *Nature (London)* 276:186–188.

181. Aghajanian GK (1982). Central noradrenergic neurons: A locus for the functional interplay between alpha-2 adrenoceptors and opiate receptors. *J Clin Psychiatry* 43:20–24.

182. Roth RH, Elsworth JD, Redmond DE (1982). Clonidine suppression of noradrenergic hyperactivity during morphine withdrawal by clonidine: Biochemical studies in rodents and primates. *J Clin Psychiatry* 43:42–46.

183. Redmond DE, Jr (1981). Clonidine and the primate locus coeruleus: Evidence suggesting anxiolytic and antiwithdrawal effects. In H Lal, S Fielding, eds. *Psychopharmacology of Clonidine.* Alan R Liss, New York, pp 147–163.

184. Redmond DE, Jr, Krystal JH (1984). Multiple mechanisms of withdrawal from opioid drugs. *Ann Rev Neurosci* 7:443–478.

185. Gold M, Redmond DE, Jr, Kleber HD (1978). Clonidine blocks acute opiate withdrawal symptoms. *Lancet* 2:599–602.

186. Gold MS, Pottash AC, Extein IL, Kleber HD (1981). Neuroanatomical sites

of action of clonidine in opiate withdrawal: The locus coeruleus connection. In H Lal, S Fielding, eds. *Psychopharmacology of Clonidine,* Alan R Liss, New York, pp 285–298.

187. Pitts DK, Marwah J (1987). Cocaine inhibition of locus coeruleus neurons. In *Problems of Drug Dependence.* NIDA Research Monograph 76. US Department of Health and Human Services, Washington, DC, pp 46–52.

188. Herz A, Teschemacher HJ, Albus K, Zieglagansberger S (1972). Morphine abstinence syndrome in rabbits precipitated by injection of morphine antagonists into the ventricular system and restricted parts of it. *Psychopharmacologia (Berlin)* 26:219–235.

189. Laschka E, Teschemacher HJ, Mehraein P, Herz A (1976). Sites of action of morphine for the development of physical dependence in rats. II. Precipitated morphine withdrawal by application of morphine antagonists into restricted parts of the ventricular system and by microinjection into various brain areas. *Psychopharmacologia (Berlin)* 46:141–147.

190. Laschka E, Herz A (1977). Sites of action of morphine involved in the development of physical dependence in rats. *Psychopharmacologia (Berlin)* 53:33–37.

191. Bozarth MA, Wise RA (1984). Anatomically distinct opiate receptor fields mediate reward and physical dependence. *Science* 224:516–517.

192. Lomax P, Ary M (1974). Sites of action of narcotic analgesics in the hypothalamus. In E Zimmerman, R George, eds. *Narcotics and the Hypothalamus.* Raven Press, New York, pp 37–49.

193. Lewis VA, Gebhart GF (1977). Evaluation of the periaqueductal central gray (PAG) as a morphine-specific locus of action and examination of morphine-induced and stimulation-produced analgesia at coincident PAG loci. *Brain Res* 124:283–303.

194. Pert C, Snyder S (1976). Opiate receptor binding-enhancement of opiate administration *in vivo. Biochem Pharmacol* 25:847–853.

195. Hitzemann R, Hitzemann B, Loh H (1974). Binding of ^{3}H-naloxone in the mouse brain: Effect of ions and tolerance development. *Life Sci* 14:2393–2404.

196. Childers SR, Simantov R, Snyder SH (1977). Enkephalin: Radioimmunoassay and radioreceptor assay in morphine dependent rats. *Eur J Pharmacol* 46:289–293.

197. Fratta W, Yang HYT, Hong J, Costa E (1977). Stability of met-enkephalin content in brain structures of morphine-dependent or footshock-stressed rats. *Nature (London)* 268:452–453.

198. Wesche D, Hollt V, Herz A (1977). Radioimmunoassay of enkephalins. Regional distribution in rat brain after morphine treatment and hypophysectomy. *Naunyn Schmiedeberg Arch Pharmacol* 301:79–82.

199. Hollt V, Przewlocki R, Herz A (1978). β-Endorphin-like immunoreactivity in plasma, pituitaries and hypothalamus of rats following treatment with opiates. *Life Sci* 23:1057–1066.

200. Bronstein DM, Akil H (1987). Effects of chronic morphine treatment on beta-endorphin immunoreactive forms in rat brain. *Soc Neurosci Abstr* 13:637.

201. Mocchetti I, Giorgi O, Schwartz JP, Fratta W, Costa E (1985). Morphine

pellets lower the hypothalamic content of proopiomelanocortin mRNA but not that of proenkephalin mRNA. *Soc Neurosci Abstr* 10:1111.

202. Ryan J, Hanig R, Schwartz J, Douglas J, Uhl GR (1987). Opiate drugs alter opioid peptide gene expression. *Soc Neurosci Abstr* 13:1003.
203. Weissman BA, Zamir N (1987). Differential effects of heroin on opioid levels in the rat brain. *Eur J Pharmacol* 139:121–123.
204. Trujillo KA, Bronstein DM, Akil H (1988). Increases in prodynorphin peptides following chronic morphine treatment. *Soc Neurosci Abstr* 14:543.
205. Hanson GR, Merchant KM, Letter AA, Bush L, Gibb JW (1987). Methamphetamine-induced changes in the striatal-nigral dynorphin system: Role of D-1 and D-2 receptors. *Eur J Pharmacol* 144:245–246.
206. Walker JM, Moises H, Coy D, Young E, Watson SJ, Akil H (1982). Dynorphin (1-17): Lack of analgesia but evidence for non-opiate electrophysiological and motor effects. *Life Sci* 31:1821–1824.
207. Walker JM, Tucker DE, Coy DH, Walker BB, Akil H (1982). Des-tyrosine-dynorphin antagonizes morphine analgesia. *Eur J Pharmacol* 85:121–122.
208. Akil H, Shiomi H, Matthews J (1985). Induction of the intermediate pituitary by stress: Synthesis and release of a non-opioid form of beta-endorphin. *Science* 227:424–426.
209. Glimscher PW, Margolin DH, Hoebel BG (1984) Neurotensin: A new 'reward peptide.' *Brain Res* 291:119–124.
210. Goldstein A (1976). Opioid peptides (endorphins) in pituitary and brain. *Science* 193:1081–1086.
211. Leslie FM (1987). Methods used for the study of opioid receptors. *Pharmacol Rev* 39:197–249.
212. Corbett AD, Paterson Sj, McKnight AT, Magnan J, Kosterlitz HW (1982). Dynorphin 1-8 and dynorphin 1-9 are ligands for the kappa-subtype of opiate receptor. *Nature (London)* 299:79–81.

CHAPTER 3

Bradykinin and Pain

Solomon H. Snyder, Donald C. Manning, and Larry R. Steranka

Introduction

Basic biomedical research attempts to understand bodily functions, but the implicit or explicit underlying assumption is that new information is being sought so as to discover more effective and safer therapies. How does molecular research into the addictive processes fit into this model? Addiction takes place to a wide variety of psychoactive substances, all of which seem to share the capacity to provide behavioral reinforcement, some enhanced sense of well-being, or euphoria. Along with their sedative effects, alcohol and barbiturates provoke euphoria in susceptible individuals. The stimulant actions of cocaine and amphetamines might in principle have therapeutic actions except for the addictive propensity associated with the euphoric actions of the drugs. Similarly, opiates, besides providing analgesia, elicit reinforcing subjective effects. The phenomena of tolerance, physical dependence, and compulsive drug-seeking behavior are common to addiction involving all of the de-pendence-producing substances. Because of the similarity in formal properties of the addictive process across different drug classes, it is conceivable that the same or closely similar general mechanism is involved in addiction to all drugs, although each utilizes distinct neuro-chemical mediators. Viewed optimistically, if one could solve the riddle of addiction to one substance, then the mystery of addiction for all classes of drugs would be revealed. From a more pessimistic vantage point, one might be concerned that most, if not all, agents that make us "feel good" seem to have abuse liability if not the capacity to cause serious addiction. In principle, sedating, antianxiety, stimulant, and central analgesic drug actions might be elicited by chemicals without provoking the enhanced sense of well-being that seems linked to abuse potential. However, up to the present time virtually all centrally acting drugs that convey these potentially therapeutic actions present addictive liabilities.

The most extensive efforts to develop nonaddicting agents are to be found in research on opiates. Many thousands of opiates have been synthesized with a view to developing nonaddicting analgesics. All sorts of theoretical principles have been utilized. Two of the most sophisticated involve the design of mixed agonist-antagonist drugs and the synthesis of chemicals that act selectively upon subtypes of opiate receptors. Thus far none of these approaches has been altogether successful. Since analgesia is one of the most important therapeutic targets in clinical medicine, one feels obliged to seek alternative strategies. The best-established non-addicting analgesics are those whose primary action is not in the central nervous system, namely the aspirin-like nonsteroidal anti-inflammatory drugs. These agents act in the periphery primarily by blocking the formation of prostaglandins. This chapter will explore another aspect of peripheral initiation of pain sensation—namely, the chemical mediator that acts upon receptors at sensory nerve endings in the periphery. The best candidate for a peripheral pain initiating substance is bradykinin.

Bradykinin, which occurs both in the brain and the periphery, may also be relevant to central mechanisms of pain perception and even of addiction. Nature often utilizes a single chemical mediator both in the central and peripheral nervous systems to serve somewhat different but closely related functions integrating an overall body response to the environment—for example, by the catecholamines norepinephrine and epinephrine. In the periphery these substances mediate the body's response to external threats by raising blood pressure, dilating the bronchial tree, and increasing the force of contraction of the heart. The norepinephrine neuronal system in the brain seems to be involved in the behavioral excitation that is also relevant to such responses. The epinephrine neuronal system in the brainstem is directly involved in the regulation of blood pressure.

Angiotensin provides another example of peripheral and central mechanisms working together toward a common goal, in this case the regulation of body salt and fluid dynamics. Acting at specific receptors in the adrenal cortex angiotensin provokes increased synthesis and release of aldosterone, thereby increasing salt retention and contributing to elevated blood pressure. Angiotensin directly constricts small blood vessels, producing pressor effects. At a variety of receptors in the brain angiotensin provokes thirst and may also play a more direct role in blood pressure regulation.

This chapter will also describe bradykinin neuronal systems in the brain, which project to sites that may be involved in coordinating pain and blood pressure responses, perhaps working in some coordinated fashion with bradykinin in the periphery, which is clearly involved in pain sensation and blood pressure regulation.

Peripheral Pain Mechanisms

A fundamental problem regarding peripheral pain transmission is identifying the initial stimulus. Plato and Aristotle speculated that pain stems from overstimulation of any of the senses. In the eleventh century

Avicenna introduced the concept that pain represents a distinct sense. Several nineteenth-century researchers utilized various spinal cord sections to distinguish between neuronal pathways conveying touch and pain inflammation.

Two related concepts that have proved crucial in understanding pain initiation are that pain is initiated by stimuli that cause tissue damage and that chemical mediators of inflammation, which attempt to repair the tissue damage, mediate pain as well as inflammation. The first of these assertions stems from observations of Henriques (1), replicated many times in succeeding years (2), that the threshold for cutaneous heat pain is about 45°C, very close to the threshold for tissue injury. The concept that the same or similar chemicals are involved in both pain and inflammation has been supported by many years of experimental evidence.

Attempting to understand chemical mechanisms of pain initiation clearly requires that we also try to comprehend mechanisms of inflammation. The inflammatory process is complex. Very briefly, tissue damage results in the release of a diverse range of substances including bradykinin, prostaglandins, leukotrienes, thromboxanes, serotonin, histamine, substance P, platelet-activating factor, and free radicals (3). These substances elicit effects associated with the inflammatory process, such as enhanced capillary permeability, allowing plasma and cellular components of blood to enter the tissue to help repair damage. Some of the substances are directly chemotactic for certain blood cells. Complex interactions occur between various inflammatory mediators. For instance, bradykinin causes mast cells to degranulate (4), releasing platelet-activating factor, which in turn releases serotonin from platelets. There are numerous other examples of such interactions.

All the inflammatory mediators have been proposed as pain-initiating substances. Although a number of them may play a role, an accumulation of evidence suggests that bradykinin is a primary mediator of pain.

Histamine

Histamine in peripheral tissues is primarily concentrated in granules within mast cells. Mast cells occur in the epiperiendoneurium in peripheral nerve and are abundant throughout connective tissue (5,6). Mast cells degranulate following various types of tissue damage, including cold and even slight pinching. Besides histamine, mast cells can release prostaglandins as well as proteolytic enzymes, which can produce bradykinin from its precursors (7).

Since the classic work of Sir Henry Dale (8), histamine has been associated with the "triple response" to tissue injury involving local reddening, a widespread flare, and finally a wheal. Pain accompanies the wheal and flare, and, since histamine reproduces the wheal and flare upon interdermal injection, histamine was proposed as a mediator of pain. A number of studies reported pain following histamine administration beneath the skin (9). However, most failed to control for the acidic pH of the histamine solution. When administered at neutral pH, histamine produces an itch but not pain (9–12). Some studies have suggested that H_1 antihistamines reduce inflammatory pain. However, these studies fail to take into consideration antihistamine effects that are unrelated to histamine receptors, such as local anesthetic actions (13). The present consensus is that antihistamines have questionable analgesic activity.

Serotonin

As already mentioned, serotonin is released from platelets by platelet-activating factor derived from mast cells. The exposure of platelets to collagen during tissue injury also releases serotonin. When applied directly to a human blister base, serotonin elicits pain (14), although its effects are substantially weaker than those of bradykinin. Serotonin also potentiates the algesic effects of bradykinin (15,16). Recently a peripheral serotonin receptor has been identified which mediates the effects of serotonin associated with pain and inflammation (14,17). These sites, designated 5-HT_3 receptors, are antagonized with considerable potency and specificity by a series of drugs that block both the direct painful effects of serotonin and the ability of serotonin to potentiate bradykinin-elicited pain on human blister base preparations.

Substance P and Calcitonin Gene-Related Peptide

Substance P is contained in nociceptive afferent fibers and is considered a neurotransmitter in the spinal cord (18,19). Substance P also is released from free nerve endings in the periphery of these sensory fibers, where it may mediate the "triple response" described above. This response apparently involves antidromic activation of adjoining terminal branches in unmyelinated fibers. Substance P released from the peripheral ends of these fibers causes vasodilatation both directly in blood vessels and indirectly by releasing histamine from mast cells (20–22). Calcitonin gene-related peptide (CGRP) has recently been identified in a substantial portion of unmyelinated sensory fibers (23,24). Since CGRP is a potent vasodilator, it may elicit effects similar to those of substance P in mediating the axon reflex.

Earlier studies had reported that substance P produces pain when injected directly into the skin. However, these preparations, prepared by extraction from natural sources, contained bradykinin (25,26). Intradermal injection of authentic substance P in humans predominantly produces itch (25).

Eicosanoids

The term "eicosanoid" refers to the physiologically active metabolites of arachidonic acid, which include the prostaglandins, thromboxanes, and leukotrienes. Eicosanoids certainly play a role in inflammation. They occur in high concentrations in inflammatory exudates (3). Of the eicosanoids, the most direct evidence for a role in pain mechanisms has been obtained for prostaglandins of the E series (PGE_1 and PGE_2) (27). In concentrations likely to be found at inflamed sites, these agents do not cause overt pain. However, they do enhance painful responses to noxious stimuli and to bradykinin (28–30). The ability of aspirin and other nonsteroidal anti-inflammatory drugs to relieve pain presumably reflects their inhibition of cyclo-oxygenase enzymatic activity with a resultant decrease in the biosynthesis of prostaglandins (31).

Bradykinin

Several lines of evidence have suggested that bradykinin is a pain mediator. This nonapeptide (Arg-Pro-Pro-Gly-Phe-Ser-Pro-Phe-Arg) is formed from the large protein precursor bradykininogen (32). Trypsin-like enzymes, collectively referred to as the kallikreins, are released along with bradykininogen into interstitial fluid following tissue damage (33).

Bradykinin is the most potent endogenous algesic substance known when tested in a variety of experimental models in humans and animals (34–37). Its effects are normally terminated rapidly by enzymatic kininase activity. However, in the acidic environment present with inflammation, kininase activity is inhibited, thereby enhancing bradykinin actions (38).

Bradykinin stimulates the synthesis and release of prostaglandins (39,40). Prostaglandins in turn potentiate the effects of bradykinin (41). This enhancement may be coupled with the potentiation of bradykinin's algesic effects by serotonin. The pain-eliciting actions of bradykinin formed during tissue injury are therefore likely to be substantially greater than those of bradykinin applied experimentally.

Bradykinin Receptor Localization

If bradykinin is a physiological stimulus to pain, its receptors should be localized to nociceptive afferent nerve fibers. Indirect evidence for such a localization has come from demonstrations that bradykinin enhances the responsiveness of nociceptive fibers (42,43). Direct evidence has come from recent autoradiographic studies.

Bradykinin receptors can be labeled with [³H]bradykinin. In smooth muscle such as guinea pig intestine, [³H]bradykinin binds with extremely high affinity, in the picomolar range (44). The properties of the receptor binding sites are consistent with the BK_2 subtype of bradykinin receptors

(45). BK_1 receptors respond selectively to bradykinin whose carboxyl terminal arginine has been removed and are not normally present in tissues but appear following tissue injury. BK_2 receptors require the intact bradykinin molecule and respond to extremely low concentrations of bradykinin. The well-characterized effects of bradykinin-stimulating phosphoinositide turnover (46,47), cyclic GMP formation (48), and contractions of smooth muscle preparations such as the guinea pig ileum and rat uterus (45) involve BK_2 sites.

To determine whether sensory neurons possess bradykinin receptors, we examined the localization of [^{3}H]bradykinin in slices of peripheral guinea pig tissues by autoradiography (49). The specificity of the binding sites was ensured by showing that [^{3}H]bradykinin associated silver grains were completely abolished by 0.1 μmol/L bradykinin and as little as 0.1 nmol/L bradykinin reduced grain density by 50%. Lysyl-bradykinin, whose affinity for receptors is similar to that of bradykinin itself, blocked receptor labeling as effectively as bradykinin. By contrast, des-Arg^9-bradykinin at 1-μmol/L concentrations had no effect on grain density and failed to influence bradykinin receptors in biochemical binding studies.

The bradykinin receptors we identified were concentrated in a narrow band in the dorsal horn of the spinal cord, the substantia gelatinosa, the dorsal root ganglion, and the dorsal root (Figure 3.1). At high-power magnification the receptor-associated grains in the dorsal root ganglion were localized to a subset of small neuronal cells most concentrated in the dorsal periphery of the ganglion. The absence of silver grains over the spinal ventral root indicates that bradykinin does not bind to all axons. Receptor-associated grains were also apparent over the sensory fibers peripheral to the dorsal root ganglion.

We also visualized bradykinin receptors in the guinea pig trigeminal ganglion and dog stellate ganglion. In the trigeminal, as in the dorsal root ganglion, grains were localized to a subset of small neuronal cells. In the stellate ganglion an intense band of silver grains was apparent over a thin, apparently unmyelinated neuronal fiber tract.

The most striking aspect of these autoradiographic studies is that bradykinin receptors are highly localized to certain sensory neurons, specifically those associated with pain transmission. Pain responses are mediated by thin, unmyelinated fibers that have small cell bodies concentrated in the periphery of the dorsal root ganglion. This description fits well with the localizations of bradykinin receptors we have observed. By contrast, touch and pressure sensation is conveyed by thick, myelinated fibers with large cell bodies in the dorsal root ganglion and terminals in relatively deep layers of the dorsal spinal cord. This restricted localization of the receptors to nociceptive neuronal fibers and cells bespeaks extraordinary specificity of physiological function.

Renal colic is an important type of clinical pain. Our autoradiograms (Figure 3.2) of the ureter reveal bradykinin receptors highly concentrated

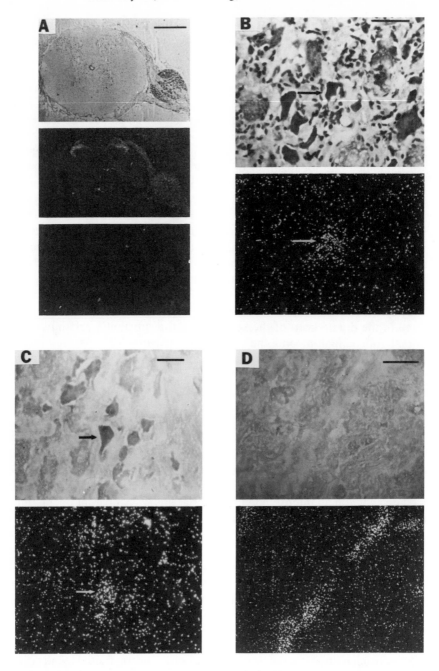

FIGURE 3.1. Autoradiographic distribution of [³H]BK receptor binding sites in guinea pig and canine primary afferent neurons. *A.* Guinea pig lumbar spinal cord and dorsal root ganglion (bar = 1 mm). (Top) Bright-field photomicrograph. (Middle) Dark-field photomicrograph from ultrafilm. Note labeling over substantia

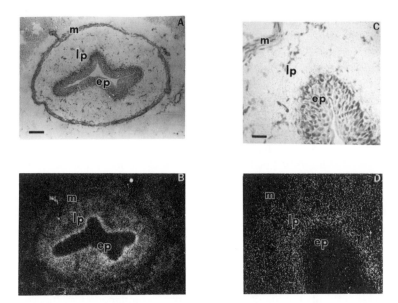

FIGURE 3.2. Autoradiographic localization of [³H]BK (0.5 nmol/L) binding in guinea pig ureter. A. Low-power bright-field photomicrograph (bar = 100 μm) of ureter cross section. B. Dark-field photomicrograph of NTB-3 emulsion-coated coverslip overlying section in A. Note the high-grain density over the lamina propria (lp) especially the subepithelial area and the relative lack of grains over the epithelium (ep) and muscle layer (M). C. High-power bright-field photomicrograph (bar = 25 μm) from A. D. Dark-field photomicrograph of C emphasizing the sharp boundary of grain density in the lamina propria at the basal layer of the epithelium and the lack of grains over the muscle layers. Adapted from Manning and Snyder (50).

gelatinosa, dorsal root, and dorsal root ganglion. (Bottom) Dark-field photomicrography of ultrafilm incubated with [³H]BK and 0.1 μmol/L unlabeled Lys-BK. B. Guinea pig dorsal root ganglion at high magnification (bar = 100 μm). (Top) Bright-field photomicrograph. (Bottom) Dark-field photomicrography from NTB3 emulsion-coated coverslip overlying the tissue section in top photo. Arrow in both photos indicates a BK-labeled dorsal root ganglion cell. C. Guinea pig trigeminal ganglion at high magnification (bar = 50 μm). (Top) Bright-field photomicrograph. (Bottom) Dark-field photomicrograph from NTB3 emulsion-coated coverslip. Arrow in both photos indicates a BK labeled cell. D. Canine stellate ganglion at high magnification, displaying both sympathetic ganglion cells and visceral afferent fibers of passage (bar = 50 μm). (Top) Bright-field photomicrograph. (Bottom) Dark-field photomicrograph from NTB3 emulsion coated coverslip. Note labeling over fiber tracts and relative absence of labeling over sympathetic ganglion cells. Adapted from Steranka et al (49).

in the subendothelial layer (50). This layer contains a dense plexus of presumably nociceptive unmyelinated fibers (51). Although it is not possible for us to establish definitively that the bradykinin receptors are localized to those fibers, there appears to be a strong likelihood. Thus these receptors may convey the pain of renal colic.

The receptor localizations we have observed may also account for pain transmission in angina. Coronary artery constriction elicits the release and accumulation of bradykinin in the coronary vasculature and myocardium (52). Epicardial administration of bradykinin stimulates cardiovascular visceral afferent nociceptors that travel to the spinal cord through the stellate ganglion (53). Clinically intractable angina is relieved by lesioning these pathways. Thus, the bradykinin receptors we have identified in nociceptive neurons in the stellate ganglion may well be associated with coronary angina pain.

Analgesic Effects of Bradykinin Antagonists

Bradykinin fulfills the major requirements of a pain mediator. It is present in damaged tissues at concentrations sufficient to cause pain (54). Highly selective receptors are specifically localized to nociceptive fibers. However, these observations do not "prove" that bradykinin actually participates in the pain elicited by tissue damage. Definitive proof requires highly selective antagonists. The situation is analogous to establishing the role of histamine in acid secretion in the stomach. Histamine was well known to stimulate acid secretion and to occur in the stomach in adequate concentrations as well as to be released from storage sites by stimuli that enhance acid secretion (55). However, for many years the gastroenterological community did not regard histamine as a physiological mediator of acid secretion. The definitive evidence came with the development of histamine H_2 antagonists.

John Stewart and colleagues synthesized thousands of bradykinin derivatives over the years. Recently they showed that certain discrete modifications conferred antagonist effects. These modifications include a substitution of D-phenylalanine at the 7 position and a replacement at the 5 and 8 positions of proline with hydroxyproline (56). More than 100 peptides related to the prototypic bradykinin antagonist structure have been synthesized. The antagonists inhibit [³H]bradykinin receptor binding in the nanomolar range and potently block the ability of bradykinin to contract the guinea pig ileum and rat uterus and to enhance phosphoinositide turnover in various tissue preparations (49). They are several orders magnitude weaker in competing at numerous other receptor binding sites. Accordingly, these agents display the potency and selectivity that would permit one to utilize them as probes to assess the physiological role of bradykinin in pain initiation.

TABLE 3.1. Antinociceptive effects of BK antagonists

A. Antagonism of acetic acid-induced writhing in mice

Treatment	Dose (μmol/kg)	Writhes
Saline		8.2 ± 0.8 (34)
NPC-349	5	4.8 ± 0.6[a] (25)
NPC-349	65	1.9 ± 0.5[a] (15)
NPC-567	10	6.1 ± 1.5 (8)
NPC-567	30	3.8 ± 0.9[a] (8)

B. Antagonism of BK- and urate-induced hyperalgesia in rat paw

Treatment	Pressure at withdrawal (g × 10^{-1})
Saline	11.1 ± 0.5 (27)
NPC-349	8.1 ± 0.4 (9)
NPC-567	9.7 ± 0.5 (18)
BK	5.9 ± 0.6[b] (17)
BK + NPC-349	11.7 ± 1.5[c] (9)
BK + NPC-567	9.5 ± 1.2 (9)
Urate	5.7 ± 0.3[b] (9)
Urate + NPC-567	8.6 ± 0.5[c] (9)

[a] Compared to saline controls using a t-test; $p < 0.05$.
[b] $p < 0.05$ [b] Compared to saline-treated rats in each experiment using Tukey's HSD test following a significant interaction term in a two-way analysis of variance; $p < 0.05$.
[c] Compared to BK- or urate-treated rats using Tukey's HSD test following a significant interaction term in a two-way analysis of variance; $p < 0.05$.

In the writhing studies (part A), mice were injected i.p. with 10 ml/kg of 0.6% acetic acid plus saline or the indicated dose of BK antagonist and writhes were recorded for a 5-minute period beginning 5 minutes after injection. Results of studies of BK- and urate-induced hyperalgesia are shown in part B. For BK hyperalgesia, rats were injected intradermally in the dorsal surface of the paw with 20 μL of saline alone or saline containing 2 nmol of BK, 20 nmol of the indicated BK antagonists, or BK plus the antagonist and tested 5 minutes later. Independent experiments were performed for each antagonist. For urate hyperalgesia, rats were injected subcutaneously (SC) in the dorsal surface of the paw with saline or 10 mg of sodium urate crystals (in 100 μL) along with saline or 200 nmol of NPC-567 (in 20 μL) and tested 4 hours later. Each of the three hyperalgesia experiments was analyzed using a separate two-way analysis of variance, and differences between means following a significant interaction term were analyzed using Tukey's HSD test. Results from the saline control and BK and NPC-567 alone groups were not different among the three experiments and were pooled after statistical analysis for presentation in the table. Values shown are the means ± SEM of the number of animals shown in parentheses. Adapted from Steranka et al (57).

TABLE 3.2. Antagonism of urate-induced hyperalgesia in rat paw by BK antagonists

Antagonist		Dose	Paw withdrawal threshold (percent of control)	
NPC No.	Sequence	(nmol/paw)	Saline	BK
567	D-Arg[Hyp^3,D-Phe^7]BK	0	100.0 ± 5.6	54.7 ± 4.5[a]
		2	92.2 ± 7.7	71.4 ± 7.5[a]
		20	88.2 ± 6.5	86.2 ± 5.1[b]
349	D-Arg[Hyp^3,Thi^{5,8},D-Phe^7]BK	0	100.0 ± 5.6	67.4 ± 3.9[a]
		2	83.9 ± 4.6	98.2 ± 4.2[b]
		20	89.9 ± 6.0	99.5 ± 10.5[b]
573	[D-Nal^1,Thi^{5,8},D-Phe^7]BK	0	100.0 ± 5.1	35.8 ± 6.9[a]
		2	103.2 ± 10.3	54.7 ± 6.4[a]
		20	103.9 ± 6.4	76.5 ± 2.8[b]
414	Lys-Lys[Hyp^{2,3},Thi^{5,8},D-Phe^7]BK	0	100.0 ± 4.6	47.2 ± 6.2[a]
		2	74.0 ± 8.1	74.5 ± 14.1[c]
		20	77.8 ± 6.2	79.9 ± 8.7[c]
722	[Leu^{5,8},Gly^6,D-Phe^7]BK	0	100.0 ± 2.9	64.7 ± 2.5[a]
		2	84.4 ± 8.5	79.8 ± 4.7[c]
		20	90.7 ± 5.6	83.0 ± 5.7[c]
566	D-Arg[Hyp^2,D-Phe^7]BK	0	100.0 ± 3.8	45.5 ± 3.7[d]
		2	87.8 ± 6.1	44.3 ± 6.4[d]
		20	93.8 ± 8.6	57.4 ± 4.1[d]

[a] Compared to saline-treated rats using Tukey's HSD test following a significant interaction in a two-way analysis of variance; $p < 0.05$.
[b] Compared to BK-treated rats following a significant interaction term; $p < 0.05$.
[c] Significant interaction term in two-way analysis of variance indicates significant ($p < 0.05$) antagonism.
[d] Compared to saline-treated rats as indicated by a significant overall BK effect with no interaction; $p < 0.05$.

Rats were injected subcutaneously into the dorsal surface of the right hind paw with saline or sodium urate crystals (10 mg in 100 μL saline) together with saline or the antagonist. The amount of pressure applied to the paw at the injection site that caused paw withdrawal was determined 4 hours after drug treatment (58). An independent experiment was run for each antagonist. In saline-treated rats, paw withdrawal occurred at 112 ± 6 grams of applied pressure. The values shown are the means of 6–10 rats. Adapted from Steranka et al (49).

The bradykinin antagonists block algesic effects of bradykinin itself in several models (49,57). More importantly, they have antinociceptive effects in several distinct animal models that predict analgesic effects in humans. For instance, in modest doses these agents antagonize acetic acid–induced writhing in mice (Table 3.1) (57). This test effectively identifies analgesic effects of opiates as well as nonopiate analgesics.

Clinical pain resulting from inflammatory tissue injury generally involves an enhanced responsiveness of pain fibers, termed "hyperalgesia." We elicited hyperalgesia by injecting urate crystals into the hind paw of rats and then applying continuously increasing pressure onto the dorsal surface of the paw with a blunt plastic rod (Table 3.2). The pressure required to cause paw withdrawal by the rats was utilized as an indication of pain threshold (58).

Several different bradykinin antagonists blocked hyperalgesia in this model. NPC-349 was the most effective antagonist, completely blocking urate effects at 2 nmol. All the other antagonists, except NPC-566, produced some inhibition of urate hyperalgesia. At 20 nmol all the derivatives produced increased effects.

In clinical gout, urate crystals are present for a substantial period of time before patients are treated with analgesics. Accordingly, we administered NPC-567 2 hours after the injection of sodium urate crystals. At the time of maximal hyperalgesia, NPC-567 (20 nmol) completely reversed hyperalgesic effects of urate (49).

Bradykinin in the Brain

Bradykinin certainly plays a role in the periphery in pain and inflammation. We wondered whether, like norepinephrine and angiotensin, there might be a central nervous system counterpart. The possibility of bradykinin systems in the brain had been explored over many years, but only circumstantial evidence could be obtained for endogenous bradykinin systems. One approach used was to evaluate the effects of injections of small doses of bradykinin intracerebrally. We were impressed by the strikingly pronounced antinociceptive effects of very small doses of bradykinin administered in the brain (59–61). Note that these effects are opposite to the nociceptive actions of bradykinin administered in the periphery. However, such paradoxically opposite effects are reminiscent of the actions of norepinephrine, which at α_2-receptors in the brain mediates hypotension, whereas at α_2-receptors in the periphery, norepinephrine provokes hypertensive responses.

Bradykinin injected peripherally is an extremely potent hypotensive agent. Indeed, the original rationale for the synthesis of the angiotensin-converting enzyme inhibitor captopril was to block the degradation of endogenous bradykinin by the enzyme. Up till the present time it is not altogether clear whether the hypotensive actions of captopril are fully attributable to blocking the formation of angiotensin II or the breakdown of bradykinin. A physiological role for bradykinin in the peripheral regulation of blood pressure is evident in the ability of the peptide bradykinin antagonists such as NPC-567 and NPC-349 to reverse the serious hypotension associated with endotoxin or hemorrhagic shock (L. Steranka, in preparation). Paradoxically, direct injections of minute doses of bradykinin in the brain have an opposite action, increasing blood pressure (62–67).

Initial attempts to identify endogenous bradykinin systems in the brain provided only indirect evidence. For instance, kallikrein, the trypsin-like enzyme that generates bradykinin, and kininase, the carboxypeptidase that degrades bradykinin, have been demonstrated in the brain (68–74). However, both kallikrein and kininase activities could be associated physiologically with peptides other than bradykinin. Bioassays involving contractile effects upon smooth muscle suggested the presence of bradykinin in brain extracts, but the specificity of such bioassays is relatively poor (68,75–77). Moreover, careful purification was not performed to rule out the possibility that substances other than bradykinin accounted for these effects.

To obtain direct evidence regarding the presence of authentic bradykinin in the brain, we first raised potent and selective antisera to bradykinin and conducted immunohistochemical mapping studies (78). The only bradykinin-containing cells observed throughout the central nervous system were in the hypothalamus. In the posterior hypothalamus a small number of cells were observed in the most dorsal portion, medial to the fields of Forel, where a few fluorescent fibers were noted. In the medial hypothalamus, the most dense collection of cells was in the dorsal area, extending from the midline to the lateral extent of the hypothalamus (Figure 3.3). A dense number of bradykinin-containing fibers emerged just dorsal to the bradykinin cells in the midline and spread over the dorsal portion of the hypothalamus. In the medial hypothalamus a large number of bradykinin-containing cells were located dorsally as were cells overlying the nucleus reuniens and zona incerta. A high density of fibers emerged from these midline cells.

Besides the very dense projection of fibers throughout the hypothalamus, the most prominent fibers were those that passed out to the lateral septal area and those that innervated the periaqueductal grey. More limited groups of bradykinin fibers extended into the cerebral cortex, especially the pyriform cortex and cingulate gyrus.

Immunohistochemical investigations cannot establish definitively that one is dealing with the authentic chemical to which antibodies have been raised. Accordingly, we purified bradykinin-like activity from rat brain extracts and established its identity as authentic bradykinin nonapeptide (79). Utilizing gel filtration chromatography as well as two reverse-phase

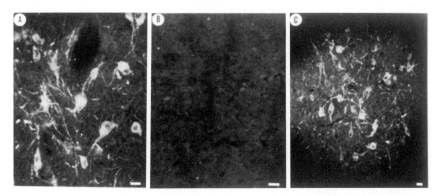

FIGURE 3.3. Immunofluorescence micrographs of bradykinin fibers and cell bodies in the dorsomedial nucleus of the hypothalamus. *A.* Immunofluorescence located in the cytoplasm of cells and extending in fibers from the perikarya. *B.* The almost complete elimination of fluorescence when the primary antisera has been preadsorbed overnight with 15 μmol/L bradykinin. *C.* Bradykinin-positive cells and fibers just lateral to the dorsomedial nucleus of the hypothalamus. Bars = 20 μm. Adapted from Correa et al (78).

HPLC systems, we could purify endogenous bradykinin extensively as well as separate it from lysyl-bradykinin and other bradykinin analogs and fragments. We established the isolated material as authentic bradykinin by several methods. First, we monitored samples by radioimmunoassay, utilizing the antibodies that had been employed for immunohistochemistry. Second, the isolated bradykinin was shown to compete for [^{3}H]bradykinin binding to receptors identically to authentic bradykinin. Finally, the isolated material behaved identically to chemically authentic bradykinin in contractile effects on the estrous rat uterus.

The regional distribution of authentic bradykinin measured by radioimmunoassay closely mirrored the distribution obtained by immunohistochemistry with levels in the hypothalamus being 8 to 10 times higher than the next highest brain regions. We could also measure levels of the large protein precursor bradykininogen by assaying bradykinin levels before and after treatment with trypsin, which converts bradykininogen to bradykinin. In the hypothalamus the apparent levels of bradykininogen were about 10 times higher than those of authentic bradykinin, whereas in whole rat brain bradykininogen levels were about 20 times higher than bradykinin concentrations. Monitoring the relative levels of bradykininogen and bradykinin under varying physiological and pathological circumstances as well as in response to drug administration may provide a means of assessing bradykinin turnover.

The localizations of bradykinin containing neurons in the brain fit with the known effects of intracerebrally administered bradykinin. When bradykinin is injected into the rat lateral ventricle, the elevated blood pressure that results is abolished by lesions of the lateral septum (62–67). Moreover, direct injections of bradykinin into the lateral septal area provoke hypertension. The discrete innervation of bradykinin fibers into the lateral septal area may well constitute the anatomical substrate for these cardiovascular effects. It is tempting to speculate that these actions, opposite to the hypotensive effects of peripherally administered bradykinin, somehow reflect a coordinated system, as has been found to be the case with the central and peripheral norepinephrine systems regulating blood pressure.

From the point of view of this discussion, most interesting is the projection of bradykinin fibers to the periaqueductal grey, where electrical stimulation is classically associated with naloxone reversible analgesia. Injections of bradykinin close to the periaqueductal grey consistently elicit analgesia (59–61). We suggest that the bradykinin fiber projections to this area are involved in these effects. Again, the fact that the effects of central and peripherally administered bradykinin obtained responses are opposite is paradoxical but tantalizing.

Conclusions

It is hard to determine whether insights into bradykinin disposition in the central nervous system and the periphery will shed light on the addictive process. The role of bradykinin in peripheral pain sensation presumably has no direct link to central mechanisms of pain appreciation that are related to drug dependence. However, the existence of bradykinin neuronal systems in the brain with seemingly reciprocal relationships to peripheral systems suggests new areas of research. Bradykinin agonist drugs that pass the blood-brain barrier might have analgesic effects. One wonders whether such agents would also produce euphoria and physical or psychological dependence. Determining whether centrally elicited strong analgesia can be provided by drugs without associated abuse liability is an important goal in pain and addiction research. Studies of bradykinin may help to address this question.

Acknowledgments. The work of this article was supported in part by USPHS grant DA-00266 and Research Scientist Award DA-00074 to S.H.S.

References

1. Henriques FC, Jr (1947). The predictability and the significance of thermally induced rate processes leading to irreversible epidermal injury. *Arch Path* 43:489–502.

2. Hardy JD, Wolff HG, Goodell H (1952). *Pain Sensation and Reactions.* Williams & Wilkins, Baltimore.

3. Moncada S, Ferreira SH, Vane JR (1978). Pain and inflammatory mediators. In JR Vane, SH Ferreira, eds. *Handbook of Experimental Pharmacology.* Springer-Verlag, New York pp 588–616.

4. Johnson AR, Erdos EG (1973). Release of histamine from mast cells by vasoactive peptides. *Proc Soc Exp Biol Med* 142:1252–1256.

5. Olsson Y (1967). Degranulation of mast cells in peripheral nerve injuries. *Acta Neurol Scand* 43:365–374.

6. Olsson Y (1968). Mast cells in the nervous system. In GH Bourne, JF Danielli, KW Jeon. eds. *International Review of Cytology.* Academic Press, Orlando, FL, pp 27–70.

7. Nennesmo I, Reinholt F (1986). Mast cells in nerve end neuromas of mice. *Neurosci Lett 69,* 296–301.

8. Dale, HH (1935). *Proc Roy Soc B* 28:319–332.

9. Lewis T, Hess W (1933). Pain derived from the skin and the mechanism of its production. *Clin Sci* 1:39–61.

10. LaMotte RH, Simone DA, Baumann TK, Shain CN, Alreja M (1987). Hypothesis for novel classes of chemoreceptors mediating chemogenic pain and itch. *Pain [Suppl]* 4:S15.

11. LaMotte RH (1989). Psychophysical and neurophysiological studies of chemically induced cutaneous pain and itch: The case of the missing nociceptor. *Progr Brain Res,* in press.

12. LaMotte RH, Simone DA, Ngeow JYF, Whitehouse J, Becerra-Cabal L, Putterman GJ (1987). The magnitude and duration of itch produced by intracutaneous injections of histamine. *Somatosensory Res* 5:81–92.

13. Hougs W, Skouby AP (1957). The analgenic action of analgetics, antihistaminics and chlorpromazine on volunteers. *Acta Pharmacol Toxicol* 13: 405–409.

14. Richardson BP, Engel G, Donatsch P, Stadler PA (1985). Identification of serotonin M-receptor subtypes and their specific blockade by a new class of drugs *Nature (London)* 316:126–131.

15. Mense S (1981). Sensitization of group IV muscle receptors to bradykinin by 5-hydroxytryptamine and prostaglandin E2.. *Brain Res* 225:95–105.

16. Hiss E, Mense S (1976). Evidence for the existence of different receptor sites for algesic agents at the endings of muscular group IV afferent units. *Pflueger Arch* 362:141–146.

17. Richardson BP, Engel G (1986). The pharmacology and function of 5-HT3 receptors. *Trends Neurosci* 9:424.

18. Lembeck F, Gamse R (1982). Substance P in peripheral sensory processes. *Ciba Found Symp* 91:35.

19. Henry JL (1976). Effects of substance P on functionally identified units in cat spinal cord. *Brain Res* 114:439–451.

20. Ebertz JM, Hirshman CA, Kettelkamp NS, Uno H, Hanifin JM (1987). Substance P-induced histamine release in human cutaneous mast cells. *J Invest Derm* 88:682–685.

21. Hagermark O, Hokfelt T, Pernow B (1978). Flare and itch induced by substance P in human skin. *J Invest Derm* 71:233–235.

22. Barnes PJ, Brown MJ, Dollery CT, Fuller RW, Heavey DJ, Ind PW (1986).

Histamine is released from skin by substance P but does not act as the final vasodilator in the axon reflex. *Br J Pharmacol* 88:741–745.

23. Brain SD, Tippins JR, Morris HR, MacIntyre I, Williams T (1986). Potent vasodilator activity of calcitonin gene-related peptide in human skin. *J Invest Derm* 87:533–536.

24. Piotrowski W, Foreman JC (1986). Some effects of calcitonin gene-related peptide in human skin and on histamine release. *Br J Derm* 114:37–46.

25. Kotani Y, Oka M, Yonehara N, Kudo T, Inoki R (1981). Algesiogenic and analgesic activities of synthetic substance P. *Jpn J Pharmacol* 31:315–321.

26. Lembeck F, Gamse R (1977). Lack of algesic effect of substance P on paravascular pain receptors. *Naunyn Schmiedeberg Arch Pharmacol* 299:295–303.

27. Ferreira SH (1985). Prostaglandin hyperalgesia and the control of inflammatory pain. In IL Bonta, MA Bray, MJ Parnham, eds. *Handbook of Inflammation: The Pharmacology of Inflammation.* Elsevier, New York pp 107–116.

28. Handwerker HO (1976). Influences of algogenic substances and prostaglandins on the discharges of unmyelinated cutaneous nerve fibers identified as nociceptors. In B Bromm, DG Albe-Fessard, eds. *Advances in Pain Research and Therapy,* vol 1, Raven Press, New York, pp 41–51.

29. Handwerker HO (1976). Pharmacological modulation of the discharge of nociceptive C fibers. In Y Zotterman, ed. *Sensory Functions of the Skin in Primates.* (Pergamon, New York, pp 427–439.

30. Handwerker HO (1976). Influences of algogenic substances and prostaglandins on the discharges of unmyelinated cutaneous nerve fibers identified as nociceptors. In JJ Bonica, D Albe-Fessard, eds. *Advances in Pain Research and Therapy,* vol 1. Raven Press, New York, pp 41–45.

31. Moncada S, Ferreira SH, Vane JR (1975). Inhibition of prostaglandin biosynthesis as the mechanism of analgesia of aspirin-like drugs in the dog knee joint. *Eur J Pharmacol* 31:250–260.

32. DiRosa M, Giroud JP, Willoughby DA (1971). Studies of the mediators of the acute inflammatory response induced in rats in different sites by carrageenan and turpentine. *J Path* 104:15–29.

33. Melmon KL, Webster ME, Goldfinger SE, Seegmiller JE (1967). The presence of a kinin in inflammatory synovial effusion from arthritides of varying etiologies. *Arthritis Rheum* 10:13–20.

34. Coffman JD (1966). The effect of aspirin on pain and hand flow responses to intra-arterial injection of bradykinin in man. *Clin Pharmacol Ther* 7:26–37.

35. Cormia FE, Dougherty JW (1960). Proteolytic activity in development of pain and itching: cutaneous reactions to bradykinin and kallikrein. *J Invest Derm* 35:21–26.

36. Guzman F, Braun C, Lim RKS (1962). Visceral pain and the pseudoaffective response to intra-arterial injection of bradykinin and other algesic agents. *Arch Int Pharmacodyn* 136:353–384.

37. Lim RKS, Miller DG, Guzman F, Rodgers DW, Wang RW, Chao SK, Shih TY (1967). Pain and analgesia evaluated by intraperitoneal bradykinin-evoked pain method in man. *Clin Pharmacol Ther* 8:521–542.

38. Edery H, Lewis GP (1963). Kinin-forming activity and histamine in lymph after tissue injury. *J Physiol* 169:568–583.

39. Juan H (1977). Mechanism of action of bradykinin-induced release of prostaglandin E. *Naunyn Schmiedeberg Arch Pharmacol* 300:77–85.

40. Lembeck F, Popper H, Juan H (1976). Release of prostaglandins by bradykinin as an intrinsic mechanism of its algesic effect. *Naunyn Schmiedeberg Arch Pharmacol* 294:69–73.
41. Hori Y, Katori M, Harada Y, Uchida Y, Tanaka K (1986). Potentiation of bradykinin-induced nociceptive response by arachidonate metabolites in dogs. *Eur J Pharmacol* 132:47–52.
42. Beck PW, Handwerker HO (1974). Bradykinin and serotonin effects on various types of cutaneous nerve fibers. *Pflueger Arch* 347:209–222.
43. Khan AA, Raja SN, Campbell JN, Hartke TV, Meyer RA (1986). Bradykinin sensitizes nociceptors to heat stimuli. *Soc Neurosci Abstr* 12:219.
44. Manning DC, Vavrek R, Stewart JM, Snyder SH (1986). Two bradykinin binding sites with picomolar affinities. *J Pharmacol Exp Ther* 237:504–512.
45. Regoli D, Barabe J (1980). Pharmacology of bradykinin and related kinins. *Pharmacol Rev* 32:1–46.
46. Yano K, Higashida H, Hattori H, Nozawa Y (1985). Bradykinin-induced transient accumulation of inositol trisphosphate in neuron-like cell line NG108-15 cells. *FEBS Lett* 181:403–406.
47. Braas KM, Manning DC, Perry DC, Snyder SH (1988). Bradykinin analogues: differential agonist and antagonist activities suggesting multiple receptors. *Br J Pharmacol* 94:3–5.
48. Snider RM, Richelson E (1984). Bradykinin receptor-mediated cyclic GMP formation in a nerve cell population (murine neuroblastoma clone N1E-115). *J Neurochem* 43:1749–1754.
49. Steranka LR, Manning DC, DeHaas CJ, Ferkany JW, Borosky SA, Connor JR, Vavrek RJ, Stewart JM, Snyder SH (1988). Bradykinin as a pain mediator: receptors localized to sensory neurons and analgesic actions of antagonists. *Proc Natl Acad Sci USA* 85:3245–3249.
50. Manning DC, Snyder SH (1986). ^{3}H-Bradykinin binding site localization in guinea pig urinary system. In LM Greenbaum, HS Margolius, eds. *Kinins IV*. Plenum, New York, pp 563–570.
51. Aung-Khin M (1973). The innervation of the ureter. *Invest Urol* 10:370–378.
52. Staszewska-Barczak J, Ferreira SH, Vane JR (1976). An excitatory nociceptive cardiac reflex elicited by bradykinin and potentiated by prostaglandins and myocardial ischemia. *Cardiovasc Res* 10:314.
53. Uchida Y, Murao S (1974). Bradykinin-induced excitation of afferent cardiac sympathetic nerve fibers. *Jpn Heart J* 15:84–91.
54. Kellermeyer RW, Graham RC (1968). Kinins-possible physiologic and pathologic roles in the man. *N Engl J Med* 279:859–866.
55. Code CF (1965). Histamine and gastric secretion: A later look, 1955–1965. *Fed Proc* 24:1311–1321.
56. Vavrek RJ, Stewart JM (1985). Competitive antagonists of bradykinin. *Peptides* 6:161–164.
57. Steranka LR, DeHaas CJ, Vavrek RJ, Stewart JM, Enna SJ, Snyder SH (1987). Antinociceptive effects of bradykinin antagonists. *Eur J Pharmacol* 136:261–262.
58. Randall LO, Selitto JJ (1957). A method for measurement of analgesic activity on inflamed tissue. *Arch Int Pharmacodyn* 111:409–418.
59. Ribeiro SA, Corrado AP, Graeff FG (1971). Antinociceptive action of intraventricular bradykinin. *Neuropharmacology* 10:725–731.
60. Corrado AP, Graeff FG, Ribeiro SA, Riccioppo Neto F (1974). Comparison of

effects of bradykinin administered intracarotideally and intraventricularly. *Cienc Cult (Sao Paulo)* 26:589–596.

61. Ribeiro SA, Rocha e Silva M (1973). Antinociceptive action of bradykinin and related kinins of larger molecular weight by the intraventricular route. *Br J Pharmacol* 47:517–528.

62. Pearson L, Lambert GA, Lang WJ (1969). Centrally mediated cardiovascular and EEG responses to bradykinin and eledoisin. *Eur J Pharmacol* 8:153–158.

63. Hoffman WE, Schmid PG (1978). Separation of pressor and antidiuretic effects of intraventricular BK. *Neuropharmacology* 17:999–1002.

64. Kondo K, Okuno T, Konishi K, Saruta T, Kato E (1979). Central and peripheral effects of bradykinin and prostaglandin E_2 on blood pressure in conscious rats. *Naunyn Schmeideberg Arch Pharmacol* 308:111–115.

65. Kariya K, Yamauchi A, Chatani Y (1982). Relationship between central actions of bradykinin and prostaglandins in the conscious rat. *Neuropharmacology* 21:267–272.

66. Lewis RE, Hoffman WE, Phillips MI (1983). Angiotensin II and bradykinin: Interactions between two centrally active peptides. *Am J Physiol* 244:R285–R291.

67. Correa FMA, Graeff FG (1975). Central site of the hypertensive action of BK. *J Pharmacol Exp Ther* 192:670–676.

68. Hori S (1968). The presence of bradykinin-like polypeptides, kinin-releasing and destroying activity in brain. *Jpn J Physiol* 18:722–787.

69. Iwata H, Shikimi T, Oka T (1969). Pharmacological significance of peptidase and proteinase in the brain (report 1)—Enzymatic inactivation of bradykinin in rat brain. *Biochem Pharmacol* 18:119–128.

70. Camagro ACM, Ramalho-Pinto FJ, Greene LJ (1972). Brain peptidase: Conversion and inactivation of kinin hormones. *J Neurochem* 19:37–49.

71. Shikimi T, Kerna R, Matsumoto M, Yamahata Y, Miyata S (1973). Studies on kinin-like substances in brain. *Biochem Pharmacol* 22:567–573.

72. Kariya K, Iwaki H, Ihda M, Maruta E, Murase M (1981). Central actions of bradykinin. I. Electroencephalogram of bradykinin and its degradation system in rat brain. *Jpn. J. Pharmacol.* 31:261–267.

73. Kariya K, Yamauchi A, Hattori S, Tsuda Y, Okada Y (1982). The disappearance of intraventricular bradykinin in the brain of the conscious rat. *Biochem Biophys Res Commun* 107:1461–1466.

74. Chao J, Woodley C, Chao L, Margolius HS (1983). Identification of tissue kallikrein in brain and in the cell-free translation product encoded by brain mRNA. *J Biol Chem* 258:15173–15178.

75. Inouye A, Kataoka K, Tsujioka T (1961). On a kinin-like substance in nervous tissue extracts treated with trypsin. *Jpn J Physiol* 11:319–334.

76. Werle E, Zach P (1970). Verteilung von Kininogen in Serum und Geweben bei Ratten und anderen Saugetieren. *Z Klin Chem* 8:186–189.

77. Pela IR, Gardy-Levassort C, Lechat P, Rocha e Silva M (1975). Brain kinins and fever induced by bacterial pyrogens in rabbits. *J Pharm Pharmacol* 27:793–794.

78. Correa FMA, Innis RB, Uhl GR, Snyder SH (1979). Bradykinin-like immunoreactive neuronal systems localized histochemically in rat brain. *Proc Natl Acad Sci USA* 76:1489–1493.

79. Perry DC, Snyder SH (1984). Identification of bradykinin in mammalian brain. *J Neurochem* 43:1072–1080.

CHAPTER 4

Neurochemical Aspects of Addiction: Opioids and Other Drugs of Abuse

A. Herz and T. S. Shippenberg

Introduction

Drugs of abuse exert marked effects on mood and motivational processes. Opioids long considered to be prototypical addictive agents produce euphoria and drug-seeking behaviors in humans and are self-administered by laboratory animals. The repeated administration of opioids and certain other drugs of abuse result in the development of tolerance and dependence. Although such latter actions are important for the maintenance of drug addiction once established, it has become increasingly apparent that they are not causal factors. Rather, there is now substantial evidence to indicate that it is the activation of endogenous reward pathways and the positive reinforcing effects produced that determine both a drug's potential for abuse and the addiction process that may subsequently ensue. Furthermore, as will be seen, the same neural system that mediates the reinforcing or motivational effects of opioids may also underlie such effects of other drugs of abuse as well as those of natural rewards.

Rewards or reinforcers are by, definition, those stimuli that establish and sustain habits by virtue of the central states they induce—states that in humans are usually associated with the subjective feeling of pleasure. A variety of animal models including both self-administration and intracranial self-stimulation have been used to determine the motivational effects of drugs of abuse. In these procedures, administration of a drug or rewarding stimulus such as electrical brain stimulation is contingent upon the performance of a specific behavioral task such as lever pressing. By evaluating drug-induced changes in performance, the ability of a drug to control behavior directly is assessed. Data so derived provide a measure of primary reinforcement processes.

Two alternative approaches that have been used to characterize drug-induced motivational effects are those of place and taste preference conditioning. In these procedures, the associations developing between the presentation of a drug and a previously neutral stimulus are examined and evaluation of a subject's behavior following presentation of the stimulus provides a measure of a drug's ability to function as a secondary reinforcer. To date, these procedures have been used to confirm the reinforcing effects of a variety of psychoactive drugs. More importantly, however, these techniques have permitted the detection of both reinforcing and aversive drug-induced motivational states and in the case of opioids have provided important new information regarding the neurochemical substrates that underlie their reinforcing as well as their dysphoric or aversive effects.

Multiple Opioid Receptors and Ligands

Since the initial discovery of the endogenous opioids (1) an increasing number of opioid peptides that contain the N-terminal sequence of either methionine-enkephalin (met-enkephalin) or leucine-enkephalin (leu-enkephalin) have been isolated. These opioid peptides originate from one of three distinct precursor molecules: Pro-opiomelanocortin (POMC), from which ACTH and α-MSH are derived, is the precursor for β-endorphin (β-EP). Met- and leu-enkephalin as well as several larger enkephalin-containing peptides including peptide E and F are derived from proenkephalin, whereas prodynorphin is a precursor for leu-enkephalin and larger peptides containing this sequence, such as dynorphin and α-neoendorphin (2). The three opioid peptide families are widely distributed throughout the neuroaxis. These peptides each have a distinct pattern of distribution within the central nervous system (CNS) (3). Of particular interest with respect to the topic of this article is the central β-EP system. Fibers that contain β-EP, originating from perikarya of the nucleus arcuatus in the mediobasal hypothalamus (MBH) (see Figure 4.12 on page 131) project to various brain regions, including limbic structures such as the ventral tegmentum and the nucleus accumbens. An additional source of this peptide is the nucleus solitarius (3). However, as will be documented here, the β-EP system originating from the MBH seems to be a key component of the neuronal circuitry mediating reward.

In addition to the multiplicity of opioid peptides, there is now ample evidence for a multiplicity of opioid receptors (4). On the basis of pharmacological experiments in whole animals, Martin et al (5) identified three distinct receptor types designated as μ, κ, and σ. Prototypic agonists at these receptor types are morphine (μ), ketocyclazocine (κ), and N-allyl normetazocine (σ). Studies employing isolated tissue preparations have shown that in addition to μ- and κ-receptors, there are also δ- and ε-receptors (6,7). The existence of opioid receptor subtypes (μ_1, μ_2, κ_1, κ_2, κ_3) has also been postulated.

Such heterogeneity has raised questions regarding the relationship between the various opioid peptides and receptor types. Morphine exhibits high affinity and selectivity for the μ-receptor. At present, however, no known endogenous opioid peptide acts selectively at this receptor type. However, some long-chain members of the proenkephalin family (eg, peptide E) have greater affinity for μ- than for either κ- or δ-receptors (2). Furthermore, although recent studies indicate the existence of opioid-alkaloids (eg, morphine) in the mammalian brain (8), it is questionable whether the small amounts detected have physiological significance. The enkephalins exhibit some selectivity for δ-receptors and, despite some activity at μ-receptors, are considered as possible endogenous ligands of this receptor type. (No compound, however, with alkaloid structure and selectivity for δ-receptors is known at the present time.) Certain prodynorphin-derived peptides bind with high affinity and selectivity to κ-receptors and may in fact be the endogenous ligands of this receptor type (2,6,9,10) In addition, several synthetic opioid ligands with a high selectivity for this receptor type (eg, U-50,488H and U-69593) have recently been described (11,12). Compounds which are specific antagonists of these particular receptor types have also been synthesized (see Table 4.1). Concerning the ε-receptor for which β-EP shows high selectivity in the rat vas deferens (7,13), there is some evidence suggesting its existence in the brain (14,15). However, β-EP also exhibits considerable affinity for μ-receptors, and it is this interaction that may mediate some of its effects in the brain (16). Finally, it is important to note that although the affinity of a ligand for the various receptor types is a major factor in determining the receptor through which it acts, the availability (ie, concentration) of a ligand at a given synapse will also govern the receptors to which it binds *in vivo* to exert its biological effects.

Motivational Properties of Opioids as Assessed by Place and Taste Conditioning

Among the various approaches used to investigate the motivational effects of drugs (see Introduction), place and taste preference condi-

TABLE 4.1. Opioid receptor-ligand relationship

Receptor type	Endogenous ligand	Exogenous ligand	Antagonist
μ	(Morphine-like alkaloid?) β-Endorphin?	Morphine DAGO	Naloxone (low dosage)
δ	Enkephalins	DPDPE	ICI 174864
κ	Dynorphin	U-50,488H U-69593	Nor-Binaltorphimine
(ε)	β-Endorphin		(β-Endorphin$_{1-27}$)

DPDPE = D-Pen^2-D-Pen^5-enkephalin; U-50,488H = (trans-3,4-dichloro-N-methyl-N(2-pyrrolidinyl)-cyclohexyl)-benzeneacetymide); U-69593 = [5α,7α8β]-(+)-N-methyl-N-[7-(1pyrrolidinyl) 1-oxa-spiro(4,5)dec-8-yl]benzenacetamide; (12) ICI 174864 = Allyl$_2$-Tyr-Aib-Phe-Leu-OH; DAGO = D-Ala^2-N-Phe^4-Gly-ol^{5}enkephalin.

tioning procedures have gained increasing interest. These classical conditioning procedures are based on the observation that animals will approach and subsequently prefer stimuli associated with appetitive reinforcers and will withdraw from or avoid those that are aversive (17,18). These procedures in contrast to operant techniques, such as self-administration and intracranial self-stimulation, have the advantage of assessing the motivational effects of substances in the drug-free state, thus circumventing the confounding of drug-induced alterations in locomotor activity with measures of reward. Furthermore, since conditioning can be obtained with as little as one stimulus pairing, the influence of such factors as tolerance and dependence upon subsequent data interpretation can be minimized (19,20).

Using these procedures it has been shown that a variety of drugs with abuse liability function as reinforcers producing conditioned place and taste preferences. A comparison of the results obtained with these and other behavioral techniques have shown that place and taste preference conditioning give only a few "false negatives" (21).

Both place and taste preference conditioning procedures have provided the first demonstrations that opioids may have reinforcing or aversive effects depending on the receptor type with which they interact (22). Figure 4.1 summarizes the results of place conditioning studies with a series of μ- and κ-opioid agonists. Administration of the μ-receptor agonists morphine, fentanyl, or sufentanyl resulted in dose-related preferences for the drug-associated place confirming that these drugs function as reinforcers in the drug-naive animal. Since the potency of these agonists in eliciting these effects parallels their differing affinity to μ-receptors (23), it can be concluded that the activation of this specific receptor type underlies their reinforcing properties. In contrast to μ-agonists, the selective κ-agonists U-50,488H and U-69593 (11,12) produced clear place aversions. Here, too, the potencies of these ligands in producing this effect correlates well with differences in their binding affinities to κ-receptors. It is also interesting to note the decreased effect of both agonists at higher doses. Although the significance of these findings remains unclear, such results may indicate an interaction of these agents with other receptor types. Similar results have also been obtained with μ- and κ-receptor agonists in taste conditioning procedures, although the doses needed to produce these effects are lower than those required for place conditioning (22).

The administration of several opioid antagonists including naloxone produce aversive effects in both place and taste conditioning procedures in rats (Figure 4.2) (20,24). Similar results were obtained in mice (25). The findings of such marked effects of an antagonist are of particular significance in that they suggest the existence of a tonically active endogenous opioid reward system, the disruption of which results in aversive states. Furthermore, since such effects are observed with doses

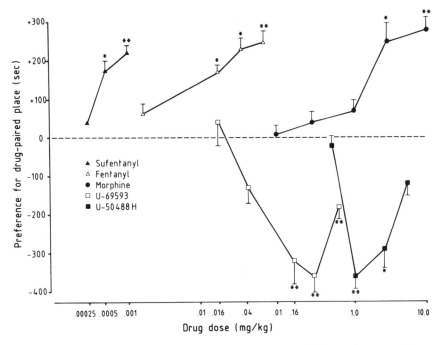

FIGURE 4.1. Place conditioning produced by the μ-opioid agonists morphine, fentanyl, and sufentanyl and the κ-opioid agonists U-50,488H and U-69593. Ordinate: mean difference (seconds) between time spent in drug- and vehicle-paired sides of the test box. Abscissa: drug dose. Points above zero indicate a place preference, points below a place aversion. Each point represents the mean conditioning score $\pm$ SEM of eight to ten rats. Asterisks denote significant place conditioning (Wilcoxon test: $*p < 0.05$; $**p < 0.01$). Adapted from Mucha and Herz (22).

of naloxone that selectively block μ-opioid receptors (16), it is suggested that this system is mediated by μ-opioid receptors. An enhancement in the motivational effect of naloxone is observed in animals that are tolerant and physically dependent on morphine (24,26). This finding is consistent with the aversive state produced by precipitated withdrawal.

Place conditioning studies investigating the motivational properties of a series of opioid mixed agonist-antagonists revealed biphasic effects of two such agents: nalbuphine and buprenorphine. Thus, whereas low doses of these opioids as a result of their high affinity and intrinsic activity at μ-receptors produced conditioned place preferences, higher doses produced place aversions. In view of the ability of these agents to interact with multiple opioid receptor types the question remained as to whether a κ-agonist or μ-antagonist action underlies their aversive effects. To address this issue place conditioning was conducted in animals

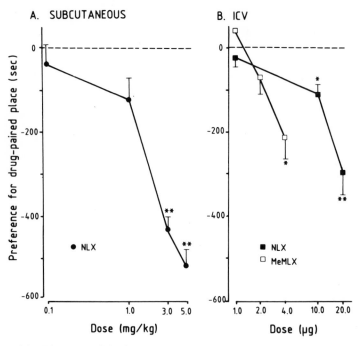

FIGURE 4.2. Place conditioning produced by subcutaneous (*A*) or intracerebroventricular (*B*) administration of opioid antagonists naloxone (NLX) and its quaternary analog methylnaloxone (MeNLX). Each point represents the mean conditioning score ± SEM of eight to ten rats. Asterisks denote significant place conditioning (*$p < 0.05$; **$p < 0.02$). From Bals-Kubik et al, in preparation.

chronically infused with a dose of naloxone sufficient to block μ- but not κ-receptors or a higher dose that blocks both receptor types. It was hypothesized that if the aversive effects of these agents resulted from an antagonism of μ-receptors, then the continual blockade of this receptor type throughout conditioning sessions should, by masking those effects associated with its acute blockade, abolish the resulting place aversions. If, however, the aversive effects of these agents were κ-receptor-mediated, no attenuation in the place conditioning should be seen. As shown in Figure 4.3, the reinforcing effect of nalbuphine (10.0 mg/kg) was abolished by μ-receptor blockade, whereas no attenuation in the aversive effects of this agent was observed. Administration of the higher naloxone dose (3.0 mg/kg/h) did, however, result in a complete attenuation of the nalbuphine-induced place aversion. This finding indicates that the aversive effect is due to a κ-agonistic and not to a μ-antagonistic property of this agent (Shippenberg et al, submitted).

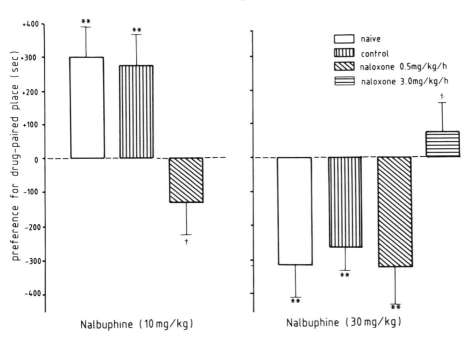

FIGURE 4.3. Influence of chronic naloxone treatment upon the biphasic motivational effects of nalbuphine. Place conditioning was evaluated in animals implanted with osmotic minipumps containing a low (0.5 mg/kg/h) or high dose (3.0 mg/kg/h) of naloxone. All conditioning and test sessions were conducted in the continual presence of the pumps. Asterisks denote significant place conditioning ($p < 0.02$); dagger (†) denotes significant effect of naloxone infusion. Administration of the low dose of naloxone, which selectively blocks μ-receptors, abolished the place preference produced by 10.0 mg/kg nalbuphine. The higher dose of naloxone abolished the place aversion induced by 30.0 mg/kg nalbuphine. From Shippenberg et al, in preparation.

Central Versus Peripheral Sites of Opioid Action

Although it is clear from the results described above that opioids have the capacity to function as reinforcing or aversive stimuli, the location of the receptor types mediating these motivational effects is still a subject of debate. Thus several studies indicate that the aversive effects observed with κ-agonists and low doses of morphine administered intraperitoneally, but not subcutaneously, are mediated peripherally via the vagus nerve (27,29). Recent experiments, however, in which the conditioning drugs were applied directly into the brain via intracerebroventricular (ICV) injections demonstrate that a cerebral site underlies both the aversive and positive reinforcing effects of opioid agonists. Thus, the ICV administration of U-50,488H and morphine at doses much lower than systemically effective levels produce conditioned place aversions and preferences, respectively (Bals-Kubik et al, submitted). Aversive effects are also observed following the ICV administration of methyl naloxone, a derivative of naloxone that does not cross the blood-brain barrier, again pointing to a cerebral locus of action (Figure 4.2).

By employing the ICV route of administration it has also been possible to examine the effects of those opioids (ie, peptides) that do not readily penetrate the blood-brain barrier after systemic application. This technique was recently used to determine the role of δ-receptors in the mediation of reward. ICV administration of the specific δ-agonist DPDPE (30) produced marked preference for the drug-associated place and the magnitude of this effect was dose-related. Pretreatment with the δ-antagonist ICI 174,864 (31), which in itself lacked reinforcing or aversive effects did not alter the reinforcing properties of μ-agonists. This antagonist did, however, abolish such properties of DPDPE (32) (Figure 4.4). Thus it is apparent that the reinforcing properties of opioids may result from an activation of either μ- or δ-receptors; this notion is also supported by data obtained from hypothalamic self-stimulation experiments (33). Further-

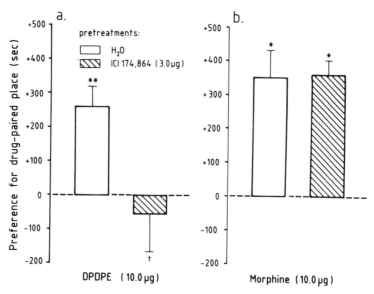

FIGURE 4.4. The influence of pretreatment with the δ-opioid antagonist ICI 174,864 upon the place conditioning produced by DPDPE (*a*) and morphine (*b*). ICI 174,864 abolished the place preference produced by DPDPE but not morphine. All drugs were injected icv. Place conditioning scores represent the mean ± SEM of six to ten rats. Asterisks denote significant place conditioning (*$p <$ 0.05; **$p <$ 0.02); dagger (†) denotes significant effect of ICI 174,864. Adapted from Shippenberg et al (32).

more, they suggest that agonists at either receptor type will have a marked potential for abuse.

Opioid Peptides and Endogenous Reward Processes: Role of β-Endorphin

The ability of opioid antagonists such as naloxone or naltrexone to induce aversive states implies the existence of one or more endogenous reward pathways, a key component of which is opioidergic in nature. The question then arises as to the identity and location of the endogenous opioidergic system involved. In view of the results with exogenous opioid agonists a role for either μ- or δ-receptor ligands, or both, must be considered.

In this context, the cerebral β-EP system originating in the MBH is of special interest. This peptide is self-administered by laboratory animals and produces conditioned place preferences following its ICV administration (34,35); Bals-Kubik et al, submitted). Moreover β-EP terminals are found in brain regions involved in the modulation of both mood and motivational processes. A role for this peptide in the actions of naloxone is suggested by the results of a recent place conditioning study that utilized bilateral radio-frequency lesions of the MBH to destroy the β-EP-containing perikarya within (36).

Such lesions resulted in a depletion of ir-β-EP in the hypothalamus and its major CNS projection sites, the septum and midbrain. This manipulation attenuated but did not abolish, the aversive effects of naloxone (36) (Figure 4.5). It did not, however, modify the effects of μ- or κ-agonists. The inability of such lesions to modify the response to μ- or κ-agonists is evidential that animals did not suffer from a generalized disruption of learning or memory processes that may have impaired their ability to acquire a conditioned response. Rather, the attenuation of the aversive effect of naloxone is most readily explained by a diminution of the release of an opioid, β-EP and a resultant decrease in the tonic activity of one or more endogenous opioidergic reward pathways.

Inasmuch as the content of other opioid peptides is affected by such lesions (37), a role for these peptides must also be considered. It is, however, unlikely that an antagonist-induced disruption of dynorphin underlies the effect of naloxone since this peptide is itself aversive (Bals-Kubik et al, submitted). Furthermore, since the blockade of δ-receptors by ICI 174,864 does not affect motivational processes, a role for enkephalins appears minimal. Thus in all probability it is the β-EP system originating from the MBH that is a key component of endogenous reward pathways, the blockade of which underlies the effects of opioid antagonists.

In line with the assumption of a role for β-EP-ergic systems in reinforcement processes are results obtained with a metabolite of β-EP

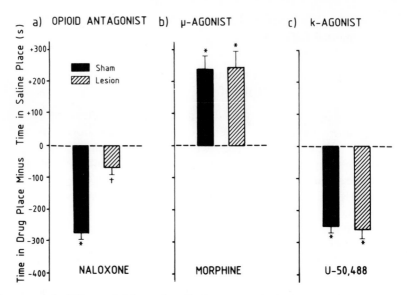

FIGURE 4.5. Effect of bilateral radio-frequency lesioning of the mediobasal hypothalamus on the motivational properties of naloxone, morphine, and U-50,488H. The aversive effect of naloxone is largely attenuated by such lesions, whereas the place preference and aversion produced by morphine and U-50,488H, respectively, are unaltered. Values represent the mean ± SEM of 8 to 12 rats. Asterisk indicates significant place conditioning ($p < 0.05$). Dagger (†) denotes significant effect of lesions. Adapted from Mucha et al (36).

known as β-EP$_{(1-27)}$. Recent studies have shown that this peptide fragment attenuates the antinociceptive effects of β-EP in mice following its ICV administration presumably by a competitive antagonism of the receptor to which β-EP binds (38,39). Place conditioning experiments in rats have also revealed an ability of β-EP$_{(1-27)}$ to antagonize the reinforcing effects of β-EP (Figure 4.6) in a dose-dependent fashion. This fragment also antagonized the reinforcing effects of selective μ- and δ-agonists but did not modify the place preference or aversion produced by respectively, the psychostimulant D-amphetamine and the κ-opioid agonist U-50,488H. Interestingly, β-EP$_{(1-27)}$, like ICI 174,864, was devoid of motivational effects, a finding that is surprising in view of its ability to block the actions of β-EP as well as μ- and δ-agonists (Bals-Kubik et al, in press).

The antagonistic activity of β-EP$_{(1-27)}$ would appear to be of functional significance since this effect is observed with physiologically relevant concentrations (40). However, the question remains as to the receptor types that underlie its antagonistic effects. Although the presence of an ε-receptor to which β-EP binds in peripheral tissues [ie, the rat vas deferens] has been demonstrated (7,13), evidence for its CNS localization

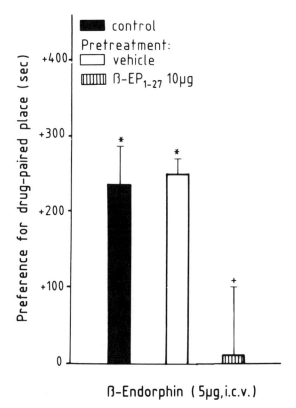

β-Endorphin (5μg,i.c.v.)

FIGURE 4.6. Antagonistic effect of β-EP$_{(1-27)}$ on the place preference induced by β-EP. β-EP$_{(1-27)}$ (10 μg icv) was administered 5 minutes prior to β-EP (5 μg icv) and was by itself devoid of any motivational effects. Columns represent the mean conditioning score ± SEM of 8–10 rats. Asterisk denotes significant place conditioning ($p < 0.05$); dagger (†) denotes significant effect of β-EP$_{(1-27)}$. From Bals-Kubik et al, *Arch Pharmacol Toxicol,* in press.

is less clear. Thus, despite autoradiographic studies indicating a distinct β-EP binding site in various forebrain areas, such as the nucleus accumbens (14,15), the high binding affinity of β-EP to both μ- and δ-sites and the ability of β-EP$_{(1-27)}$ to antagonize ligands acting at either receptor type preclude definitive statements concerning the receptor types mediating their motivational effects.

Endogenous Opioidergic Tone: Role of μ-, κ-, and δ-Receptor Ligands

The aversion produced by the opioid antagonist, naloxone, is most readily attributable to an antagonism of opioid receptors that, even in the absence of a rewarding stimulus, are tonically activated. Naloxone exhibits an approximately 10 times higher binding affinity to μ- than either δ- or κ-receptors (6). Therefore, in view of the effectiveness of low doses in producing place aversions, it is likely not only that the blockade of μ-receptor underlies its aversive effects but also that the activation of this receptor is required for the maintenance of neutral motivational states. Furthermore, the lack of effect of ICI 174,864 in place conditioning indicates that, although δ-receptors are involved in the reinforcing properties of exogenous opioids, they are not crucial for the expression of naloxone's aversive effects (32). Only preliminary data regarding the effects of κ-opioid receptor blockade are available: pilot studies with norbinaltorphimine, a putative κ-receptor antagonist (41) have revealed place preferences in some animals following ICV injections. However, a clear dose-response relationship is lacking, and the results at present are only of borderline significance (Bals-Kubik et al, submitted). A limited selectivity of norbinaltophimine for κ-receptors was found *in vivo* in contrast to *in vitro* (42).

In summary, the results of studies with several opioid antagonists suggest the existence of a tonically active μ-opioidergic reward pathway, which may counterbalance the aversive effects of κ-receptor activation. Whether there is a tonic activity of κ-receptors of a magnitude equal to that of μ-receptors remains unclear.

Factors that Modify the Reinforcing and Aversive Effects of Opioids

It is becoming increasingly apparent that the motivational effects of endogenous and exogenous opioids may change under certain conditions. Of particular interest are recent findings showing an altered response to opioids in an animal model of chronic pain. In Sprague-Dawley rats suffering from monoarthritis (induced by injection of Freund's adjuvant into the hind limb) κ-agonists were ineffective in producing place aversions, whereas no significant alterations in the reinforcing effects of the μ-agonist (morphine) were observed (Shippenberg et al, in press). These data may be interpreted in a rather simplistic (and anthropomorphic) manner; thus, in conditions of chronic pain, the analgetic effects of drug can oppose and thus compensate for aversive affective states that would normally ensue (Figure 4.7). This phenomenon is of interest in view of the fact that there is limited evidence as to whether κ-opioids induce analgesia in the clinical sense and do not just inhibit nociceptive reflexes.

Do changes also occur in the motivational effects of opioids following their repeated administration? In animal models of opioid self-administration, tolerance is rarely encountered. Although tolerance to the euphorigenic effects of opioids have been described, there are also reports that addicts maintain a relatively constant intake over time. In

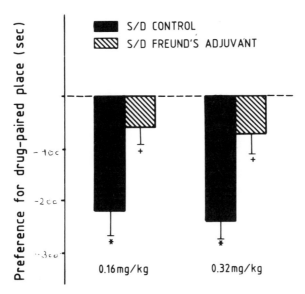

FIGURE 4.7. Reversal of the aversive effects of the selective κ-opioid agonist U-69593 in chronic arthritic rats (Freund's adjuvant). Columns represent the mean conditioning score ± SEM of eight to ten rats. Asterisk denotes significant place conditioning ($p < 0.05$); dagger (†) denotes significant difference between control and arthritic rats. Shippenberg et al, *Pain*, in press.

recent experiments we found that pretreatment of rats for 4 days with relatively low doses of morphine (5.0 mg/kg/12 h) shifted the dose response curve for morphine- or fentanyl-induced place preference to the right, whereas the aversion induced by the κ-receptor ligand U-69593 was not changed (Figure 4.8). In contrast, pretreatment with U-69593 induced tolerance to the aversive effect of this drug but did not affect the morphine preference. Place preferences induced by amphetamine were unchanged by pretreatment with either opioid agonist. Thus these data demonstrate that in a classical conditioning model selective tolerance develops to both the reinforcing and aversive properties of opioids whereas no cross-tolerance occurs between μ- and κ-opioid receptor induced motivational effects (43).

Involvement of Endogenous Opioids in the Motivational Effects of Other Drugs

Lithium is the drug of choice in the treatment of mania and the prophylaxis of bipolar affective disorders, and there are some indications that an opioidergic mechanism underlies its motivational effects. The

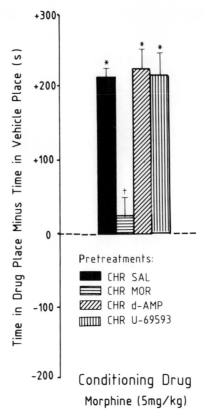

FIGURE 4.8. Influence of chronic opioid agonist or D-amphetamine treatment upon place conditioning produced by morphine. Rats received SC injections of either saline, morphine, U-69593, or D-amphetamine for 4 days prior to conditioning. Columns represent the mean conditioning score ± SEM of eight to ten rats. Asterisk denotes significant place conditioning ($p < 0.05$); dagger (†) denotes significant chronic treatment effect. Adapted from Shippenberg et al (43).

acute administration of lithium in humans may produce aversion and dysphoria. This agent also produces aversive effects in rats as assessed by place preference conditioning (22). Chronic infusion of naloxone at a dose that inactivates μ- but not κ-receptors throughout the duration of conditioning abolishes the effect of lithium indicating that its aversive action results from an antagonism of μ-receptors. As observed with naloxone, lesions of the MBH which deplete ir-β-EP in the CNS also abolish the aversive effect of lithium (44) (Figure 4.9). These data and those showing a selective effect of chronic lithium treatment upon the motivational effects of μ-opioid receptor ligands (44) indicate an involvement of both β-EP and μ-receptors in mediating at least one component of lithium's actions and are in line with previous data indicating an interaction

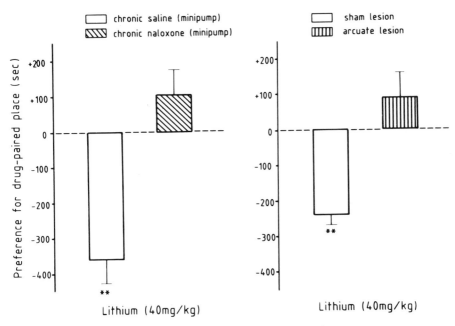

FIGURE 4.9. Influence of μ-receptor blockade or bilateral radio-frequency lesions of the MBH upon the aversive effects of lithium. *Left:* Rats were implanted with osmotic minipumps containing water or a dose of naloxone, which blocks μ- but not κ-receptors. All conditioning sessions were conducted in the continual presence of the pumps. *Right:* Rats received sham lesions or bilateral radio-frequency lesions of the MBH, 1 week prior to conditioning. Each column represents the mean score $\pm$ SEM of eight to ten rats. Asterisks denote significant place conditioning ($p < 0.01$); Adapted from Shippenberg et al (44).

between opioids and this ion (46). As such these data also support the hypothesis that a disruption in the basal activity of endogenous opioidergic systems may underlie certain affective disorders.

Activation of Endogenous Opioids by Other Rewards

In the previous animal models discussed, the effects of exogenous drugs upon opioidergic systems were investigated. There is also direct evidence that endogenous opioids may play a role in other affective behaviors. Thus, the phenomenon of stress-induced analgesia and its (at least) partial blockade by naloxone indicate that endogenous opioid peptides are released in stressful situations (47). There are also indications that opioid peptides play a key role in positively motivated rewarding situations. Non–food-deprived rats expecting or receiving highly desirable food (candy, chocolate milk) exhibited an increase in nociceptive thresholds that could be antagonized by naloxone (48). In the hypothalamus of such rats β-EP levels were significant reduced (but dynorphin levels were unchanged). A decrease in opioid receptor specific binding sites in hypothalamus, but not in other brain areas was also observed (Figure 4.10). These results indicate a release of β-EP in the hypothalamus in response to palatable food (49) and indicate that opioid peptides are released in the brain not only in stressful but also in rewarding situations. Furthermore, it is clear that β-EP plays a particular role in this emotional response (50).

Experience in Humans

The motivational properties of morphine and other opioids that are agonists at μ-receptors in humans requires no further elaboration (see Introduction). Respective data concerning the effects of selective δ-receptor ligands are not, however, available. In the case of κ-opioid receptor ligands, a study in human volunteers in which psychiatric rating scales were used to evaluate emotional and conceptual experiences showed that injection of a benzomorphan derivative with preferential κ-receptor agonist activity (MR 2033) elicited dose-dependent dysphoric

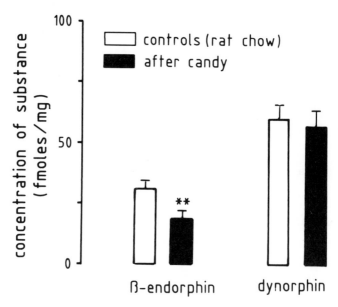

FIGURE 4.10. Concentration of β-EP and dynorphin in the hypothalamus of nondeprived rats that received a highly preferred food (candy: hatched columns) or rat chow (controls: open columns) to eat during a 20-minute period. Data represent the mean ± SEM of 10–23 rats per group. Asterisks indicates a significant difference (p < 0.01) from controls. Adapted from Dum et al (49), with permission, copyright 1983, Pergamon Journals Ltd.

and psychotomimetic effects, which were antagonized by naloxone (51). These data indicate that not only σ-receptors but also κ-opioid receptors mediate psychotomimesis. It may be suggested that these effects are equivalent to the aversion observed in the place conditioning procedure in rats.

Naloxone (preferentially acting at μ-receptors) as well as κ-opioid agonists produce aversive effects in rodents. There are also several reports describing aversive effects of naloxone in (opioid-naive) humans (52–55). Taken as a whole, the symptomatology seems to be rather mild, and in some cases there were no symptoms at all (56,57). The reason for such species differences is not quite clear. It may be that in the case of humans the occupation of opioid receptors with endogenous ligands in the test situation is lower than that in rats (and mice). In this context it is also interesting to note that, in monkeys, naloxone functions as a negative reinforcer in the absence of opioid dependence (58,59).

Links Between Opioids and Dopamine in Motivational Processes

Findings of an attenuation in the reinforcing effects produced by electrical brain stimulation and certain drugs of abuse following the administration of dopamine (DA) receptor antagonists have suggested an involvement of dopaminergic systems in reinforcement processes (60,61). If, however, dopaminergic neurons are a critical component of those tonically active pathways subserving reward, then the blockade of DA receptors or an inhibition of DA release should, as observed with naloxone, induce aversive states. Furthermore, if the DA hypothesis of reward is correct, such manipulations should also abolish the reinforcing effects of all drugs of abuse including those of opioids. Until recently, however, such effects have not been evident. Thus the DA antagonists pimozide, haloperidol, and α-flupentixol are ineffective in producing place or taste aversion (62–65) and do not function as negative reinforcers in other paradigms. Similarly, although there have been reports of an attenuation in the reinforcing property of opioids by neuroleptics or 6-OHDA lesions, such effects are variable and in some cases lacking (66,67).

The identification of two distinct DA receptor types (D_1, D_2) within the CNS (68) and the availability of antagonists selective for each have offered the possibility to reevaluate the dopamine hypothesis of reward and the involvement of D_1 versus D_2 receptors in the mediation of reinforcing and aversive states (62,63). Acute administration of the selective D_1 antagonist SCH-23390 caused clear conditioned place aversions, whereas the D_2 antagonists sulpiride and spiperone as well as the mixed D_1-D_2 antagonist haloperidol lacked such effects. Such findings provide apparent support for the hypothesis that there is a tonic activation of D_1 but not D_2 receptors, the disruption of which results in aversive states.

Figure 4.11 shows the influence of D_1 receptor blockade upon the motivational properties of morphine as assessed by place preference conditioning. As can be seen, the continual blockade of D_1 receptors throughout conditioning sessions abolished the reinforcing effect of morphine. Blockade of D_2 receptors by $(-)$sulpiride and spiperone, however, was without effect. An attenuation in the reinforcing effects of intracranial self-stimulation and psychostimulants by D_1 receptor blockade has also been reported (69,70). Together such findings indicate that the rewarding effects of a variety of stimuli result from a stimulation of DA release and an increase in D_1 receptor activation.

Does a decrease in dopamine transmission and a subsequent reduction in the tonic activity of D_1 receptors underlie the aversive effects of opioids? If such is the case then the chronic infusion of a D_1 antagonist during conditioning should, by the continuous inactivation of this recep-tor type, mask any drug-induced decreases in D_1 receptor stimulation and result in an attenuation of those effects that are mediated by this mechanism. Chronic treatment with a D_1 antagonist abolished the aver-

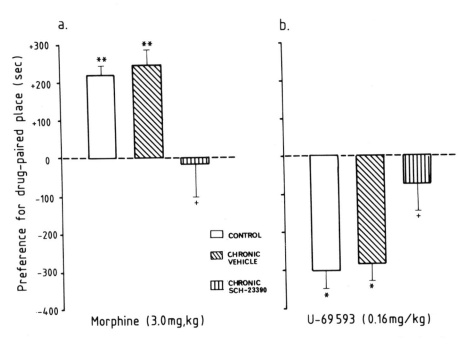

FIGURE 4.11. Effect of chronic D_1 receptor blockade on the motivational properties of morphine and U-69593. Rats were implanted with osmotic mini-pumps containing the selective D_1 receptor antagonist SCH 23390 or vehicle. Columns represent the mean conditioning score $\pm$ SEM of eight to ten rats. Asterisks denote significant place conditioning (*$p < 0.05$; **$p < 0.02$); dagger (†) indicates significant effect of SCH 23390. Adapted from Shippenberg and Herz (62).

sive effects of both a κ opioid agonist (Figure 4.11) and a low dose of the opioid antagonist naloxone, whereas D_2 antagonists were without effect (63). Thus, as shown in Table 4.2, it would appear that D_1 receptors are critical for the expression of reinforcing as well as aversive states.

Identification of the Brain Dopamine Reward Pathway Subserving Opiate Reward

The use of microinjection techniques has permitted the identification of specific brain regions involved in the reinforcing properties of opioids. Both self-administration and place conditioning studies have revealed that the injection of morphine or enkephalin analogs into several brain areas, including the lateral hypothalamus, septum, ventral tegmentum (VTA) and nucleus accumbens is reinforcing (70–74). Although such results demonstrate that an opiate action in these areas is *sufficient* for reward, they do not permit the delineation of which action is *necessary* for reward. However, the recent findings (73) that both the rate of acquisition and doses producing reinforcement are lowest in the VTA suggest that this site may be of critical importance. This conclusion receives additional support from studies showing that the reinforcing effects of intravenously administered heroin are attenuated by injections of a hydrophilic opioid antagonist into the VTA (75). Microinjections of methyl naloxonium into the nucleus accumbens, a major projection site of the VTA, but not other brain areas, were also effective (76). Thus it would appear that an activation of opioid receptors located on neurons in both these areas plays a critical role in opioid reward. It is important to note that the rewarding action of morphine in the VTA is not associated with physiological dependence—that is, with symptoms of withdrawal following the discontinuation of opioid administration (74). Hence positive rather than negative reinforcing effects of opioids underlie their abuse potential. Whether or not the same brain regions underlying reinforcement are also involved in mediating the aversive effects of opioids is unknown and, as yet, has not been investigated.

As is apparent from the preceding paragraphs, both the VTA and nucleus accumbens appear to be critically involved in the reinforcing actions of opioids. These regions are also key components of the mesolimbic DA system, the perikarya of which are located in the VTA (77). As such, this dopaminergic pathway would appear to be a primary target upon which opioidergic ligands act to exert their reinforcing effects.

There are several lines of evidence suggesting that the interaction between opioid and DA systems occurs in the VTA (73,78–80). First, this region is innervated by β-EP fibers originating in the MBH as well as by those containing dynorphin and enkephalin (3), as shown in Figure 4.12. The presence of D_1 and D_2 receptors is also well documented (81). Secondly, place conditioning studies have revealed that 6-OHDA lesions

TABLE 4.2. Dopaminergic transmission relationship

Motivation				
Increase = reward	Morphine Enkephalins β-Endorphin Amphetamine Cocaine	μ = receptors δ = receptors ε = receptors	Increase of DA release	Activation of D_1 receptors
Decrease = aversion	U-50,488H	κ-receptors	Decrease of DA release	Inactivation of D_1 receptors
	Naloxone SCH23390	μ =, δ = receptors		
No effect	Spiperone (−) Sulpiride			Blockade of D_2 receptors

This table summarizes the apparent relationship between DA pathways and rewarding and aversive drug-induced motivational states. As can be seen, opioids as well as psychostimulants increase DA release. It is postulated that this increase and the subsequent stimulation of D_1 receptors underlies their rewarding properties. In contrast, drugs which induce aversive effects either decrease DA release or inactivate D_1 but not D_2 receptors. Blockade of D_2 receptors does not change motivation.

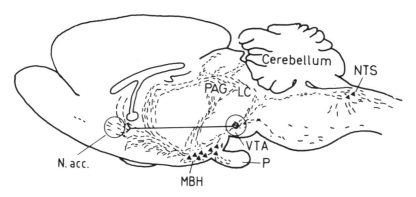

FIGURE 4.12. Schematic representation of the cerebral β-EP system and its putative connections with DA pathways ascending from the midbrain (VTA). The major portion of the cerebral β-EP system arises from perikarya located in the mediobasal hypothalamus (MBH) and projects from there to many parts of the brain, in particular the diencephalon and midbrain. A few of the β-EP fibers originate in the nucleus tractus solitarius (NTS). Thus fibers make connections with the DA system originating in the ventral tegmental area (VTA) and ascend to mesolimbic areas including the nucleus accumbens (n.acc.). P = pituitary.

which deplete DA in the VTA attenuate the reinforcing effect of heroin (64), and a recent study using the self-administration paradigm has shown that such lesions also block the acquisition of intravenous heroin self-administration (82). In the latter study, an impairment of learning processes can be discounted since subjects with similar lesions learned to perform an operant response for food reinforcement.

If this dopaminergic system is activated by reward, then an increase in DA release should be evident in response to those opioids that function as reinforcers. Indeed, unilateral microinjections of morphine into the VTA induce contralateral rotation, indicative of an increase in dopaminergic neurotransmission (83). Furthermore the firing rates of DA containing cells in this region are increased by either systemic or microiontophoretic applied morphine (84). Direct evidence for an increase in DA release has been obtained by examining neurochemical changes in response to morphine. Employing the technique of *in vivo* dialysis, Imperato and DiChiara (85) have reported an increase in DA release in the nucleus accumbens, the termination site of many VTA fibers. Studies assessing levels of 3-methoxytyramine, which provides a more indirect index of DA release, have also provided evidence for a stimulatory effect of morphine (84).

Data regarding the role of the mesolimbic DA system in mediating the aversive action of opioids is lacking. However, in view of the apparent involvement of DA (and specifically the D_1 receptor) in both the reinforcing and aversive effects of opioids, it may be suggested that μ- and

κ-agonists act at the same dopaminergic substrate, but exert opposing effects. Thus whereas μ- (and possibly δ-agonists) increase DA release, κ-agonists inhibit this release. There is, in fact, some indication for this possibility. *In vivo* release experiments have shown that in contrast to morphine, the κ-agonist, U-50,488H produced an inhibition of DA release in the nucleus accumbens (85). Such findings are also in line with the location of presynaptic opioid receptors on dopaminergic fibers originating from the VTA. Nevertheless, other sites and mechanisms of action of κ-agonists must be considered and their investigation represents an area of research that has not been explored.

Mechanisms of Reinforcement of Other Addictive Drugs

From the previous sections, it is evident that the primary, if not the only, site of action of opioids in regard to their reinforcing effects is the ascending mesolimbic dopaminergic system. This system is also activated by such psychostimulants as amphetamine and cocaine and underlies their reinforcing effects. Thus 6-OHDA lesions of the nucleus accumbens as well as neurotoxic lesions of the DA-ergic cell bodies of the VTA block the acquisition and maintenance of amphetamine self-administration (74,86,87). A disruption in DA-ergic neurotransmission also abolishes the place preferences induced by amphetamine and cocaine (64,88). In addition, microinjections of psychostimulants or DA directly into the nucleus accumbens are rewarding. The involvement of the D_1 receptor in such actions is also suggested by the finding that D_1 receptor blockade abolishes the self-administration of amphetamine as well as its reinforcing effects as assessed by place preference conditioning (69,89).

The question must still be raised, however, as to whether those neuronal elements in the mesolimbic system enacted upon by psychostimulants are those upon which opioids act. The finding that animals injected with morphine into the VTA decrease their intake of systemically administered cocaine (82) suggests that, indeed, such is the case. Thus although these drugs of abuse initially activate different components of the mesolimbic system (opioids activate the DA-ergic cell bodies in the VTA and psychostimulants activate the DA-ergic terminal field in the nucleus accumbens), the net result is an increase in DA-ergic neurotransmission in the nucleus accumbens. It is this action that appears to be crucial for the perception of reward.

Other drugs of abuse include sedative-hypnotics such as ethanol, the benzodiazepines, and weak psychostimulants such as nicotine and caffeine (90). Although less is known about the mechanisms by which these drugs exert their motivational effects, evidence suggests an involvement of DA-ergic neurons and specifically the mesolimbic system. Thus ethanol, nicotine, and caffeine have been shown to increase DA release in the nucleus accumbens (DiChiara et al, personal communication), and

4. Neurochemical Aspects of Addiction

6-OHDA lesions of this region abolish the reinforcing effects of the benzodiazepine diazepam (91). Ethanol has also been shown to interact with the endogenous opioid system (92) and thus may directly or indirectly via its actions in the VTA activate the DA system. Although much additional research is needed, including studies in which the localization of the reward-relevant receptors for each of these drugs is examined, the existing data is compatible with the hypothesis that all drugs of abuse activate the mesolimbic DA system, which is the final common pathway subserving reward.

Comparisons Between Opioids and Other Drugs of Abuse

Drugs of abuse have in common the ability to function as reinforcers, an effect that is fundamental to the initiation of drug use. In addition, however, as shown in Table 4.3, there are significant differences between them that may be of importance for the understanding of the addiction process:

1. The mechanism of activation of the mesolimbic system by these agents differs. Thus it is not clear in which way the effects of opioids and sedative hypnotics, which generally have inhibitory actions at the cellular level, activate the DA pathway (presynaptic action? interneurons?). Opioids have depressant properties at other brain structures. Depending on the species, dosage, or time after application, these depressant or sedative actions may even predominate and mask the psychomotor stimulation brought about by the activation of the DA system (93).
2. The prolonged administration of opioids (and sedative-hypnotics) induces physical dependence as indicated by the pronounced withdrawal syndrome associated with the cessation of drug intake. In the case of psychostimulants such an effect is lacking or, if it occurs, is much less marked. The "rebound" effects observed after psychostimulant discontinuation are not considered to be expressions of real physical dependence, comparable to those effects seen after opioids (90). In view of the lack of physical dependence in response to psychostimulants, it must be concluded that dependence is not a major factor that contributes to the acquisition of drug-taking behavior. It may, however, play an important role in the continuation of compulsive drug use. In this regard, it would be predicted that the termination of psychostimulant abuse would be easier than that of other substances.
3. The ability of opioids in contrast to psychostimulants to produce physical dependence indicates that those adaptive mechanisms leading to this phenomenon occur in opioidergic as opposed to dopaminergic pathways. Furthermore, it suggests that with regard to opioids the processes underlying reinforcement and dependence are separable. Indeed, this has been shown in recent studies. Thus in morphine-dependent

TABLE 4.3. Psychomotor stimulant theory of addiction

		Motivation	DA transmission	Tolerance	Physical dependence
Opioids	$\mu = \delta$ = receptor ligands	Reward	↗	+	+
	κ = receptor ligands	Aversion	↙	+	+
Psychomotor stimulants	Amphetamine	Reward	↗	+	−
	Cocaine	Reward	↗	(+)	−
'Depressants'	Alcohol	Reward	(↗)	+	+ +
	Barbiturates	Reward	(↗)	+	+ +
	Benzodiazepines	Reward	(↗)	+	+

This table summarize similarities and differences in the effects of opioids and CNS stimulants and depressants. It is important to note that all drugs of abuse function as reinforcers and increase DA neurotransmission in the nucleus accumbens. They do not all, however, induce tolerance and/or dependence.

rats, withdrawal symptomatology can be precipitated by local injections of naloxone into the periventricular and periaqueductal gray regions. On the other hand, no withdrawal symptomatogy is observed following naloxone administration into the VTA (94–96).

4. Tolerance develops after the repeated administration of opioids as well as psychostimulants. However, its development is not directly related to the initation of the addictive processes. Indeed, tolerance may develop after the continuous intake of centrally acting drugs such as anticholinergics, antidepressants, neuroleptics etc (90), which are devoid of rewarding properties. On the other hand, it has been shown that tolerance develops to the rewarding effects of opioids (43). This indicates that drug effects on "psychic" phenomena are not in principle different from those seen in somatic functions. Such a pharmacological view is supported by the fact that the aversive properties of opioids are also subject to the development of tolerance.

Concluding Remarks

Twenty years ago Dole and Nyswander (97) speculated that addiction may represent a type of metabolic disease and in 1976 Goldstein (98) postulated that a genetic hypofunction of an endogenous reward system could be a predisposing factor leading to narcotic addiction. There is now ample indication for the existence of at least one endogenous reward system, represented by the mesolimbic dopaminergic pathway and, as pointed out here, β-EP seem to play an important role in maintaining the tonic activity of this system.

Stress as well as pleasure can activate this reward system. These emotions also have the capacity to affect the perception of pain, thereby indicating a functional interaction between those pathways subserving motivational and pain processes (99). In view of the ability of β-EP to modulate responses to pain and stress at the sensory as well as the affective level, the perception of reward, and appetitively motivated behaviors, it can be suggested that it is the β-endorphinergic system that plays a decisive role in the integration of these actions.

Finally, it is apparent that a functional disruption of endogenous reward pathways, by a blockade of the actions of β-EP, can induce aversive and/or dysphoric states. Prior to the introduction of specific antidepressants, the so-called Opium Kur was widely used in the treatment of endogenous depression (100). Since that time, there have been several attempts to use synthetic opioids for the same purpose (101,102). Despite encouraging results, the risk of dependence development prevented a broader application of this treatment (interestingly, however, the development of addiction is not mentioned in older reports concerning the Opium Kur). The hypothesis, however, of a connection between depression and the activity of endogenous opioidergic reward mechanism is supported by data indicating an involvement of opioidergic mechanisms in the pharmacological actions of lithium (see above). Further investigations along this line may provide new insights into the physiological and pathological significance of endogenous opioid systems in the control of mood and motivation as well as drug use and its abuse.

Acknowledgment. This work was supported by Bundesgesundheitsamt, Berlin.

References

1. Hughes I, Smith TW, Kosterlitz, HW, Fothergill LA, Morgan BA, Morris, HR (1975). Identification of two related pentapeptides from the brain with potent opioid agonist activity. *Nature (London)* 258:277–279.
2. Höllt V (1986). Opioid peptide processing and receptor selectivity. *Ann Rev Pharmacol Toxicol* 26:59–77.
3. Watson SJ, Akil H, Khachaturian H, Young E, Lewis, ME (1984). Opioid systems: Anatomical, physiological and clinical perspectives. In J Hughes, HOJ Collier, MJ Rance, MB Tyers, eds. *Opioids: Past, Present and Future.* Taylor and Francis, London, pp 145–178.
4. Zukin RS, Zukin SR (1984). The case for multiple opiate receptors. *Trends Neurosci,* May: 160–164.
5. Martin WR, Eades CG, Thompson JA, Huppler RE, Gilbert PE (1976). The effects of morphine- and nalorphine-like drugs in the nondependent and morphine-dependent chronic spinal dog. *J Pharmacol Exp Ther* 197:517–532.
6. Paterson SE, Robson LE, Kosterlitz HW (1984). Opioid peptides. In S Udenfriend, J Meienhofer, eds. *The Peptides,* vol. 6, *Opioid Peptides,* Academic Press, Orlando, FL pp 147–189.
7. Schulz R, Wüster M, Herz A (1981). Pharmacological characterization of the ε-opiate receptor. *J Pharmacol Exp Ther.* 216:604–606.
8. Weitz CJ, Lowney LI, Faull KF, Feistner G, Goldstein, A (1986). Morphine and codeine from mammalian brain. *Proc Natl Acad Sci USA* 83:9784–9788.
9. Chavkin C, James IF, Goldstein A (1982). Dynorphin is a specific endogenous ligand of the κ-receptor. *Science* 215:413–415.
10. Wüster M, Schulz R, Herz A (1979). Highly specific opiate receptors of dynorphin-(1-13) in the mouse vas deferens. *Eur J Pharmacol* 62:235–236.
11. VonVoigtlander PF, Lahti RA, Ludens JH (1983). U 50,488H: A selective and structurally novel non-mu (kappa) opioid agonist. *J Pharmacol Exp Ther* 224:7–11.
12. Lahti RA, Mickelson MA, McCall JM, VonVoigtlander PF (1985). [³H]-69593: A highly selective ligand for the opioid κ receptor. *Eur J Pharmacol* 109:281–284.
13. Garzón J, Schulz R, Herz A (1985). Evidence for the ε-type of opioid receptor in the rat vas deferens. *Molec Pharmacol* 28:1–9.
14. Goodman RR, Houghten RA, Pasternak GW (1983). Autoradiography of [³H]β-endorphin binding in brain. *Brain Res* 288:334–337.

15. Houghten RA, Johnson N, Pasternak GW (1984). [^{3}H]-β-endorphin binding in rat brain. *J Neurosci* 4:2460–2465.
16. Millan MJ, Członkowski A, Herz A (1987). Evidence that μ-opioid receptors mediate midbrain 'stimulation produced analgesia' in the freely moving rat. *Neuroscience* 22:885–896.
17. Capell H, LeBlanc AE, Endrenyi L (1973). Aversive conditions by psychoactive drugs: Effects of morphine and chlordiazepoxide. *Psychoparmacology* 29:239–246.
18. Kumar R (1972). Morphine dependence in rats: Secondary reinforcement from environmental stimuli. *Psychopharmacology* 60:59–65.
19. Mucha RF, van der Kooy D, O'Shaughessy M, Bucenieks P. (1982). Drug reinforcement studied by the use of place conditioning in rat. *Brain Res* 243:91–105.
20. Mucha RF, Iversen SD (1984). Reinforcing properties of morphine and naloxone revealed by conditioned place preferences: A procedural examination. *Psychopharmacology* 82:241–247.
21. Swerdlow NR, Gilbert D, Koob GF (1988). Conditioned drug effects of spatial preference: critical evaluation. AA Bulton, GB Baker, A Greenshaw, eds. *Neuromethods,* vol 13, *Psychopharmacology I.* Human Press, Clifton, NJ, in press.
22. Mucha RF, Herz A (1985). Motivational properties of kappa and mu opioid receptor agonists studied with place and taste preference conditioning. *Psychopharmacology* 86:274–280.
23. Magnan J, Paterson SJ, Tavani A, Kosterlitz HW (1982). The binding spectrum of narcotic analgesic drugs with different agonist and antagonist properties. Naunyn Schmiedeberg's *Arch Pharmacol* 319:197–205.
24. Stolerman IP, Pilcher CWT, D'Mello GD (1978). Stereospecific aversive property of narcotic antagonists in morphine-free rats. *Life Sci* 22:1755–1762.
25. Mucha RF, Walker MJK (1987). Aversive property of opioid receptor blockade in drug-naive mice. *Psychopharmacology* 93:483–486.
26. Mucha RF (1987). Is the motivational effect of opiate withdrawal reflected by common somatic indices of precipitated withdrawal? A place conditioning study in the rat. *Brain Res* 418:214–220.
27. Bechara A, van der Kooy D (1985). Opposite motivational effects of endogenous opioids in brain and periphery. *Nature (London)* 314:533–534.
28. Bechara A, Zito KA, van der Kooy D (1987). Peripheral receptors mediate the aversive conditioning effects of morphine in the rat. *Pharmacol Biochem Behav* 28:219–225.
29. Bechara A, van der Kooy D (1987). Kappa receptors mediate the peripheral aversive effects of opiates. *Pharmacol Biochem Behav* 28:227–233.
30. Cotton R, Kosterlitz HW, Paterson SJ, Rance MJ, Traynor JR (1985). The use of ^{3}H-[D-Pen^2,D-Pen^5] enkephalin as a highly selective ligand of the δ-binding site. *J Pharm Pharmacol* 84:927–932.
31. Cowan A, Zhu XZ, Porreca F (1985). Studies in vivo with ICI 174, 864 and [D-Pen^2, D-Pen^5] enkephalin. *Neuropeptides* 5:311–314.
32. Shippenberg TS, Bals-Kubik R, Herz A (1987). Motivational properties of opioids: evidence that an activation of δ-receptors mediates reinforcement processes. *Brain Res* 436:234–239.
33. Jenck F, Gratton A, Wise RA (1987). Opioid receptor subtypes associated

with ventral tegmental facilitation of lateral hypothalamic brain stimulation reward. *Brain Res* 423:34–38.

34. Van Ree JM, Smyth DG, Colpaert FC (1979). Dependence creating properties of lipotropin C-fragment (β-endorphin): evidence for its internal control of behavior. *Life Sci* 24:495–502.

35. Amalric A, Cline AEJ, Martinez JL, Bloom FE, Koob GF (1987). Rewarding properties of β-endorphin as measured by conditioned place preference. *Psychopharmacology* 91:14–19.

36. Mucha RF, Millan MJ, Herz A (1985). Aversive properties of naloxone in non-dependent (naive) rats may involve blockade of central β-endorphin. *Psychopharmacology* 86:281–285.

37. Millan MJ, Millan MH, Przewłocki R (1984). Lesions of the hypothalamic arcuate nucleus modify discrete brain and pituitary pools of dynorphin in addition to β-endorphin in the rat. *Neurosci Lett* 48:149–154.

38. Nicolas P, Li CH (1985). β-Endorphin$_{(1-27)}$ is a naturally occurring antagonist to etorphine-induced analgesia. *Proc Natl Acad Sci USA* 82:3178–3181.

39. Hammonds RG, Nicolas P, Li CH (1984). Endorphin(1-27) is an antagonist of β-endorphin analgesia. *Proc Natl Acad Sci USA* 81:1389–1390.

40. Zakarian S, Smyth D (1979). Distribution of active and inactive forms of endorphins in rat pituitary and brain. *Proc Natl Acad Sci USA* 76:5972–5976.

41. Portoghese PS, Lipkowski AW, Takemori AE (1987). Binaltorphimine and nor-binaltorphimine, a potent and selective κ-opioid receptor antagonist. *Life Sci* 40:1287–1292.

42. Birch PJ, Hayes AG, Sheehan MJ, Tyers MB (1987). Norbinaltorphimine: antagonist profile at κ opioid receptors. *Eur J Pharmacol* 144:405–408.

43. Shippenberg TS, Emmett-Oglesby MW, Ayesta FJ, Herz A (1988). Tolerance and selective cross-tolerance to the motivational effects of opioids. *Psychopharmacology,* in press. 96:110–115.

44. Shippenberg TS, Millan MJ, Mucha RF, Herz A (1988). Involvement of β-endorphin and μ-opioid receptors in mediating the aversive effects of lithium in the rat. *Eur J Pharmacol,* 154:135–144.

45. Shippenberg TS, Herz A (1988). Influence of chronic lithium treatment upon the motivational effects of opioids. *Eur J Pharmacol,* in press.

46. Stengaard-Pederson K, Schou M (1982). In vitro and in vivo inhibition by lithium of enkephalin binding to opiate receptors in the brain. *Neuropharmacology* 21:817–823.

47. Akil H, Young E, Walker JM, Watson SJ (1986). The many possible roles of opioids and related peptides in stress-induced analgesia. *Ann NY Acad Sci* 467:140–153.

48. Dum J, Herz A (1984). Endorphinergic modulation of neural reward systems indicated by behavioural changes. *Pharmacol Biochem Behav* 21:259–266.

49. Dum J, Gramsch C, Herz A (1983). Activation of hypothalamic β-endorphin pools by reward induced by highly palatable food. Pharmacol. Biochem. Beh. *18,* 443–447.

50. Dum J, Herz A (1987). Opioids and Motivation. Interdisciplinary Science Rev.. *12,* 180–190.

51. Pfeiffer A, Brantl V, Herz A, Emrich HM (1986). Psychotomimesis mediated by κ opiate receptors. Science *233,* 744–776.

52. Hollister LE, Johnson K, Boukhabza D, Gillespie HK (1981). Aversive

effects of naltrexone in subjects not dependent on opiates. *Drug Alc Depend* 8:37–41.

53. Jones RT, Herning R (1979). Naloxone-induced mood and physiologic changes in normal volunteers. In E Usdin, WE Bunney, NS Kline, eds. *Endorphins in Mental Health Research*. Macmillan, New York, pp 484–491.

54. Grevert P, Goldstein A (1977). Effects of naloxone on experimentally induced ischemic pain and on mood in human subjects. *Proc Natl Acad Sci USA* 74:1291–1294.

55. Crowley TJ, Wagner JE, Zerbe G, MacDonald M (1985). Naltrexone-induced dysphoria in former opioid addicts. *Am J Psychiatry* 142:1081–1084.

56. Grevert P, Goldstein A (1978). Endorphins: Naloxone fails to alter experimental pain or mood in humans. *Science* 199:1093–1095.

57. Malcolm R, O'Neil PM, Von JM, Dickerson PC (1987). Naltrexone and dysphoria: A double-blind placebo controlled trial. *Biol Psychiatry* 22:710–716.

58. Downs DA, Woods JH (1976). Naloxone as a negative reinforcer in rhesus monkeys: Effects of dose, schedule, and narcotic regimen. *Pharmacol Rev* 27:397–405.

59. Hoffmeister F, Wuttke W (1973). Negative reinforcing properties of morphine antagonists in naive rhesus monkeys. *Psychopharmacologia* 33:247–258.

60. Wise RA, Bozarth MA (1982). Action of drugs of abuse on brain reward systems: an update with specific attention to opiates. *Pharmacol Biochem Behav* 17:239–243.

61. Wise RA (1987). The role of reward pathways in the development of drug dependence. *Pharmacol Ther* 35:227–262.

62. Shippenberg TS, Herz A (1987). Place preference conditioning reveals the involvement of D_1-dopamine receptors in the motivational properties of μ- and κ-opioid agonists. *Brain Res* 436:169–172.

63. Shippenberg TS, Herz A (1988). Motivational effects of opioids: influence of D_1 versus D_2 receptor antagonists. *Eur J Pharmacol* 151:233–242.

64. Spyraki C, Fibiger HC, Phillips AG (1982). Dopaminergic substrates of amphetamine-induced place preference conditioning. *Brain Res* 253:185–193.

65. Mackey WB, Van der Kooy D (1985). Neuroleptics block the positive reinforcing effects of amphetamine but not of morphine as assessed by place conditioning. *Pharmacol Biochem Behav* 22:101–105.

66. Van Ree JM, Ramsey N (1987). The dopamine hypothesis of opiate reward challenged. *Eur J Pharmacol* 134:239–243.

67. Fibiger HC (1978). Drugs and reinforcement mechanisms: a critical review of the catecholamine theory. *Ann Rev Pharmacol Toxicol* 18:37–56.

68. Creese I, Sibley DR, Hamblin MW, Leff SE (1983). The classification of dopamine receptors: Relation to radioligand binding. *Ann Rev Neurosci* 6:43–74.

69. Koob GF, Le HT, Creese I (1987). The D_1 dopamine receptor antagonist SCH 23390 increases cocaine self-administration in the rat. *Neurosci Lett* 79:315–320.

70. Nakajima S, McKenzie GM (1986). Reduction of the rewarding effect of brain stimulation by blockade of dopamine D_1 receptor with SCH 23390. *Pharmacol Biochem Behav* 24:919–923.

71. Phillips AG, LePiane FG (1980). Reinforcing effects of morphine microinjection into the ventral tegmental area. *Pharmacol Biochem Behav* 12:965–968.
72. Olds ME (1982). Reinforcing effects of morphine in the nucleus accumbens. *Brain Res* 237:429–440.
73. Bozarth MA, Wise RA (1983). Neural substrates of opiate reinforcement. *Progr Neuropsychopharmacol* 7:569–575.
74. Goeders NE, Lane JD, Smith JE (1984). Self-administration of methionine enkephalin into the nucleus accumbens. *Pharmacol Biochem Behav* 20:451–455.
75. Britt MD, Wise RA (1983). Ventral tegmental site of opiate reward: Antagonism by a hydrophillic opiate receptor blockade. *Brain Res* 258:105–108.
76. Vaccarino FJ, Corrigall WA (1987). Effects of opiate antagonist treatment into either the periaqueductal grey or nucleus accumbens on heroin-induced locomotor activation. *Brain Res Bull* 19:545–549.
77. Fibiger HC, Philips AG (1986). Reward, motivation, cognition: psychobiology of mesotelencephalic dopamine systems. *Handbook of Physiology* Sect 1. *The Nervous System* vol. 4. *Intrinsic Regulatory Systems of the Brain*. Baltimore: Williams & Wilkins, pp 647–675.
78. Stinus LS, Koob GF, Ling N, Bloom F, LeMoal M (1980). Locomotor activation induced by infusion of endorphins into the ventral tegmental area: evidence for opiate-dopamine interactions. *Proc Natl Acad Sci USA* 77:2323–2327.
79. Jackson D, Schenk JO, Kalivas PW (1987). Enkephalin in the A10 region increases dopamine release in the nucleus accumbens as assessed by the in vivo voltametry. *Soc Neurosci Abstr* 13:1305.
80. Latimer LG, Duffy P, Kalivas PW (1987). Mu-opioid receptors involvement in enkephalin activation of dopamine neurones in the ventral tegmentum area. *J Pharmacol Exp Ther* 241:328–337.
81. Boyson SJ, McGonigle P, Molinoff PB (1986). Quantitative autoradiographic localization of the D_1 and D_2 subtypes of dopamine receptors in rat brain. *J Neurosci* 6:3177–3188.
82. Bozarth MA, Wise RA (1986). Involvement of the ventral tegmental dopamine system in opioid and psychomotor stimulants. In LS Harris, ed. *Problems of Drug Dependence, 1985*. US Government Printing Office, Washington DC, pp. 242–248.
83. Holmes L, Bozarth MA, Wise RA (1983). Circling from intracranial morphine applied to the ventral tegmental area in rats. *Brain Res Bull* 11:295–298.
84. Wood PL (1983). Opioid regulation of CNS dopaminergic pathways: A review of methodology, receptor types, regional variations and species differences. *Peptides* 4:595–601.
85. Imperato A, Di Chiara G (1985). Opposite effects of μ and κ opiate agonists on dopamine release in the nucleus accumbens and caudate of freely-moving rats. *Br J Pharmacol* 86:532.
86. Lyness WH, Friedle NM, Moore KE (1979). Destruction of dopaminergic nerve terminals in nucleus accumbens: Effects of D-amphetamine self-administration. *Pharmacol Biochem Behav* 11:553–556.
87. Pettit HO, Ettenberg A, Bloom FE, Koob GF (1984). Destruction of

dopamine in the nucleus accumbens selectively attenuates cocaine but not heroin self-administration in rats. *Psychopharmacology* 84:167–173.

88. Morency MA, Beninger RJ (1986). Dopaminergic substrates of cocaine-induced place conditioning. *Brain Res* 399:33–41.

89. Leone P, Di Chiara D (1987). Blockade of D-1 receptors by Sch 23390 antagonises morphine and amphetamine-induced place preference conditioning. *Eur J Pharmacol* 135:251–254.

90. Jaffe JH (1985). Drug addiction and drug abuse. In A Goodman, A Gilman eds. *The Pharmacological Bases of Therapeutics,* 7th ed. Macmillan, New York, pp. 532–581.

91. Spyraki C, Fibiger HC (1988). A role for the mesolimbic dopamine system in the reinforcing properties of diazepam. *Psychopharmacology* 94:133–137.

92. Hoffman PL, Chung CT, Tabakoff B (1984). Effects of ethanol, temperature and endogenous regulatory factors on the characteristics of striatal opiate receptors. *J Neurochem* 43:1003–1010.

93. Van der Kooy D, Mucha RF, O'Shaughnessy M, Bucenieks P (1982). Reinforcing effects of brain microinjections of morphine revealed by conditioned place preference. *Brain Res* 243:107–117.

94. Wei E, Loh HH, Way EL (1972). Neuroanatomical correlates of morphine dependence. *Science* 17:616–617.

95. Laschka E, Teschemacher HJ, Mehraein P, Herz A (1976). Sites of action of morphine involved in the development of physical dependence in rats. II. Morphine withdrawal precipitated by application of morphine antagonists into restricted parts of the ventricular system and by microinjection into various brain areas. *Psychopharmacology* 46:141–147.

96. Bozarth MA, Wise RA (1984). Anatomically distinct receptor fields mediate reward and physical dependence. *Science* 224:516–517.

97. Dole VP, Nyswander ME (1967). Heroin addiction—A metabolic disease. *Arch Intern Med* 120:19–24.

98. Goldstein A (1976). Opioid peptides (endorphins) in pituitary and brain. *Science* 193:1081–1086.

99. Herz A, Millan MJ, Shippenberg TS (1988). Cerebral opioid systems in pain modulation and motivational processes. NIDA Research Monograph, in US Department of Health and Human Services, Washington, DC.

100. Herz A, Emrich HM (1983). Opioid systems and the regulation of mood: Possible signficance in depression. In J Angst, ed. *The Origins of Depression: Current Concepts and Approaches.* Dahlem Konferenzen. Springer-Verlag, Berlin, pp 221–234.

101. Emrich HM (1984). Endorphins in psychiatry. *Psychiat Develop* 2:97–114.

102. Emrich HM, Vogt P, Herz A (1982). Possible antidepressant effects of opioids. Action of buprenorphine. *Ann NY Acad Sci* 398:108–112.

CHAPTER 5

Which Molecular and Cellular Actions of Ethanol Mediate Reinforcement?

Floyd E. Bloom

Introduction

There are now several accepted CNS actions of ethanol obtainable with doses that reflect the human self-administration range. Actions at the molecular level include disordering of membrane lipids, functional alterations in membrane proteins, ion channels, and second-messenger-generating regulatory proteins, and changes in the metabolism of neurotransmitters. Actions at the cellular level include alterations in effectiveness of neurotransmitter actions, alterations in the effectiveness of specific neuronal pathways, and alterations in the spontaneous, or environmentally regulated activity of large arrays of neurons. This chapter reviews some of these molecular and cellular actions in an attempt to determine whether any "vertically linked" series of actions can yet be sufficiently aligned with the reinforcing behavioral action of alcohol to suggest the mechanisms that mediate such reinforcement.

Over the past decade, there has been a resurgence of interest in analysis of the intoxicating and dependence-forming actions of ethanol (1). Most of the work described in this chapter has been directed at the questions of how and where ethanol may act on the brains of experimental animals to produce the behavioral phenomena and neurological dysfunctions known colloquially as intoxication. Recent research at the cellular level has suggested several consistent effects of ethanol within a blood alcohol concentration range that may be regarded as meaningful for human intoxication, including alterations in effectiveness of neurotransmitter actions, alterations in the effectiveness of specific neuronal pathways, and alterations in the spontaneous or environmentally regulated activity of large arrays of neurons. Given the hierarchical relationships between levels of inquiry in the chemical, physiological, and behavioral disciplines that comprise the field of alcohol research, meaningful insight into mechanisms requires a form of vertical reasoning that is often applied to medical problems (2).

In this presentation I will briefly review data from an ongoing investigation of the cellular electrophysiology of ethanol intoxication (3–5) and augment these data with other cellular and molecular effects of ethanol on the central nervous system (CNS) that have been reported by others. Following the specific instructions of our convener, Dr. Goldstein, I will then seek to determine whether a usefully heuristic case could be assembled that might favor one or more of these effects as the mediative mechanisms underlying the behavioral reinforcing effects of ethanol. I might note in passing, that it was at Dr. Goldstein's urging that I first participated in the molecular, cellular, and behavioral world of drugs of abuse (6), and that in many ways it was his forceful presence in the field of opioid pharmacology that led to the strategies and data described here.

My colleagues and I first pursued the early cellular effects of ethanol on the cerebellar cortex (7) and within the hippocampal formation (8) as model systems partly because the major neuronal circuitry and neurotransmitters operating within these two known ethanol-sensitive brain regions were already well established when we began, and partly because the functions of those regions may be readily assumed to represent sensitivity to ethanol. Those initial studies have been heuristic beyond expectation. The results of the studies of ethanol in the cerebellum then led to two other brain regions, both known to project to the cerebellar cortex: the nucleus locus ceruleus and the inferior olivary complex.

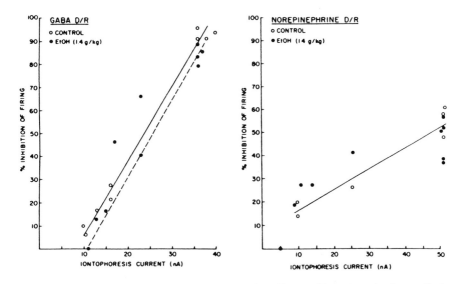

FIGURE 5.1. Derived dose-response curves for effects of iotophoretically applied norepinephrine and GABA on cerebellar Purkinje neurons, showing lack of change in effectiveness of either transmitter between control and ethanol treatment. Based on unpublished observations of Siggins and Staunton; see Bloom et al (9).

Ethanol Actions on Cerebellar Neurons

The initial studies suggested that rat Purkinje neurons were relatively resistant to locally applied ethanol (up to 3 mol/L) but did respond to systemic injections of ethanol, in doses that produced far lower local tissue concentrations—for example, 25–100 nmol/L (9). The response consisted of a major change in Purkinje discharge pattern: an increased frequency of the climbing fiber bursts, with modest increases in modal intervals of single-spike firing (9). In keeping with the relatively unchanged single-spike firing patterns, we observed (Figure 5.1) no shift in dose-response effectiveness of the transmitters γ-aminobutyric acid (GABA), norepinephrine, glutamate, or serotonin (9).

Climbing fiber bursts reflect the activity of the neurons from which climbing fibers arise—namely, neurons of the inferior olivary nucleus. Thus, the apparent activation of olivary neurons by systemic ethanol, and our earlier and less extensive evidence of resistance to direct effects of ethanol on Purkinje neurons favor the interpretation that the acute intoxicating effects of ethanol on cerebellar and vestibular function do not arise through actions at the synaptic level within the cerebellar cortex.

Effects of Ethanol on Inferior Olivary Neurons

Despite our observations of a significant time-dependent and dose-dependent increase in climbing fiber-mediated bursts, precisely the opposite effect was then reported by others (10,11) after acute ethanol; that is, there was a significant decline in climbing fiber-mediated Purkinje cell bursts. After considerable additional experiments, we can now attribute these differences to the different anesthetics and routes of ethanol administration employed in the two studies (Figure 5.2). We have therefore concluded that the most likely effect of ethanol on the inferior olivary complex under conditions that approximate the unanesthetized state is an increased firing rate, in turn derived from the synchronous discharge of the olivary neurons (8,12).

The mechanism by which ethanol causes olivocerebellar activation remains unclear. Of the several possibilities considered (12), an indirect mediation of this effect by some metabolite of ethanol, such as a harmaline-like β-carboline (formed by condensation of acetaldehyde and serotonin), is an attractive possibility that might explain why systemic ethanol elevates cerebellar Purkinje cell (8) and inferior olivary neuron activity (12), whereas locally applied ethanol has negligible depressant or transiently depressant effects on unit activity (7,13).

Indeed, it is well known that the rodent inferior olivary complex exhibits dense 5-HT-containing fibers, ending in apparent perineuronal terminals on large neurons of the olive (14). We confirmed these findings

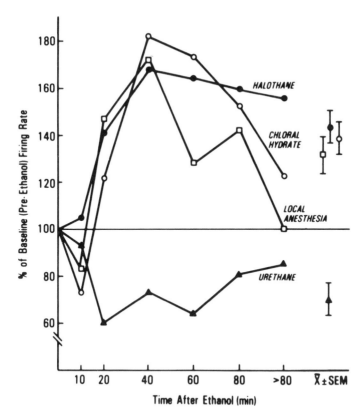

FIGURE 5.2. Effects of 2 g/kg intraperitoneal ethanol on inferior olive neurons under the various anesthetic conditions. The data are expressed as percent of the pre-ethanol baseline firing rate, averaged over all cells studied at the given time epochs. Data points with error bars at far right of the graph are overall means = SEM for firing-rate changes after ethanol. Local anesthesia does not differ significantly from chloral hydrate or halothane ($p < 0.05$), but does from urethane ($F = 25.04$, $p < 0.05$). Modified from Siggins et al (4).

(15) and then tested whether this innervation by 5-HT neurons participates in the actions of ethanol on olivary cells, comparing the effects of ethanol in normal rats and in rats that had been pretreated intracisternally or intracerebroventricularly with the 5-HT specific toxin, 5,7-dihydroxytryptamine (16). We observed in studies combining electrophysiology followed by 5-HT immunocytochemistry (15) that after this treatment, reduction in the number of 5-HT immunoreactive terminals was consistently linked to loss of the ability of systemic ethanol to activate olivary neuron firing. This result is compatible with, but clearly does not prove, the possibility that the intact 5-HT innervation, firing and releasing 5-HT during exposure to ethanol, could permit production of a 5-HT-β-carboline–like metabolite.

F.E. Bloom

Effects of Ethanol on Locus Ceruleus Neurons

One of the inferences of our early cerebellar studies (8) was that during the period of withdrawal from chonic exposure to ethanol, the neurons of the locus ceruleus should become hyperactive. We therefore turned our attention directly to these neurons (17). To measure ethanol action we followed the several specific functional properties that we had observed for these neurons in unanesthetized, freely behaving rats (18,19) and squirrel monkeys (20). After baseline characteristics were determined, ethanol was injected in cumulative doses to evaluate dose-related changes.

Ethanol had no significant effect on the mean spontaneous discharge rates of locus ceruleus neurons at any dose range between 0.5 and 3.0 g/kg, intraperitoneally, nor did the drug alter either latency or reliability of the response of locus ceruleus (LC) neurons to antidromic stimulation. However, as shown in Figure 5.3, there was a pronounced

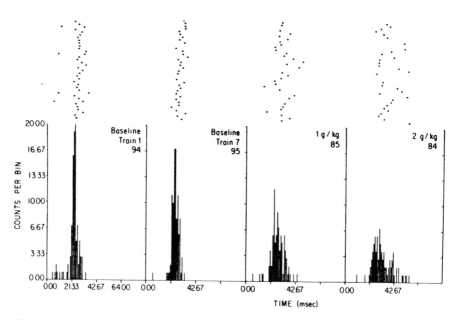

FIGURE 5.3. Poststimulus histogram responses of a single rat LC neuron following single-peripheral-nerve electrical stimuli. Above each panel are shown the "raster" displays on a time axis similar to the histograms below. Each dot represents the time at which the first orthodomic spike was recorded following the peripheral stimulus at just suprathreshold levels. Two preethanol (baseline) panels and two postethanol panels are shown. Note that the rather precise latency in the baseline periods is made extremely variable following the ethanol administration. Reprinted by permission from *Nature* 1982; 296:857–860. Copyright © 1982 Macmillan Magazines Ltd.

dose-dependent depression by ethanol ($p < 0.0005$, $n = 11$) when these same LC neurons were evaluated for their response to a standardized orthodromic sensory stimulus (17).

Significant effects of ethanol were observed at even lower blood levels when the orthodromic sensory responses of LC neurons were evaluated for the fidelity of the response latency. Ethanol increased substantially the variations in trial-to-trial response latencies for single tests of sensory responsiveness. When several indices of the variations in afferent activation were evaluated statistically (17), the greatest magnitude effect and lowest ethanol dose effect was related to the standard deviation of the response latencies (significantly increased at 0.5 g/kg; maximal effect: 325% increase at 3 g/kg). Possibly, the increased variability of orthodromic sensory response latency may be associated with a second sensitive action of ethanol on LC neurons observed in our study—namely, an increase in the inhibitory period that follows antidromic activation.

This effect of ethanol and the LC could be considered as a major detriment to normative function and a possible mechanism mediating intoxication (3,9). Locus ceruleus neurons have a highly divergent trajectory and produce potent and specific forms of conditional actions on their target neurons (21,22). Although LC actions appear to be inhibitory when tested on the basal discharge properties of their cortical target neurons, the effect also enhances or enables those targets to respond more effectively when the targets are driven by other afferents (excitatory or inhibitory) that may be simultaneously active. Given the phasic discharge of the LC neurons in the awake, behaviorally responsive rat, we have suggested (21,23) that the LC system can bias its targets to favor phasic adaptation to unexpected external environmental stimuli. Significant alteration of the normal precise sensory responses of the LC would, under this view, significantly disrupt the ability of specific external sensory stimuli to elicit appropriate adaptive responses as confirmed behaviorally (22). Expressed more simply, ethanol-induced disruption of locus ceruleus sensory responsiveness may be expected to alter cortical information processing, and may thus be a basis for further investigation of how ethanol intoxication is produced.

More recently, Pineda, Neville, and Foote (24) in our Alcohol Research Center examined squirrel monkeys, trained to sit in a chair and to respond to frequent or infrequent auditory cues while EEG was recorded from chronically implanted screw electrodes. They observed (24) that squirrel monkeys can generate a rate-positive complex cortical wave when infrequent auditory cues are presented. The amplitude of this response was found to be inversely proportional to the frequency of the eliciting cue and exhibited trial-to-trial sequential dependencies. Following bilateral electrolytic locus ceruleus lesions (the loss of ascending neocortical noradrenergic fibers was confirmed by immunohistochemistry) the amplitude of the late positive complex was markedly diminished. The effects of locus ceruleus lesions are thus similar in some respects to the effects of ethanol on locus ceruleus firing.

In Vivo Studies: Hippocampal Pyramidal Cells

The hippocampal pyramidal cell (HPC) has also proven to be a fruitful testing ground for ethanol effects. Extracellular recordings *in vivo* indicate that systemically administered ethanol alters hippocampal EEGs and multi-unit and single-unit firing rates, as well as field potential and single unit responses evoked by stimulation of afferent inputs (4,13). Although most of these studies found depressant effects (usually at high supraintoxicating doses of ethanol), we have noted (25) that systemic ethanol also can facilitate both excitatory and inhibitory responses to certain afferent stimulation.

To determine whether one or more of the endogenous hippocampal transmitters might be involved in the enhancement by ethanol of the excitatory and inhibitory afferent pathways, we tested the effect of ethanol on the responses of identified pyramidal cells to iontophoretically applied transmitters in the halothane-anesthetized rat.

Systemic ethanol at doses chosen to yield blood ethanol levels of about 80 or 150 mg% markedly enhanced excitatory responses to iontophoresis of acetylcholine (ACh) in CA1 or CA3 pyramidal cells over ten rats, within 15 minutes after injection of ethanol. The effect reached a peak at about 30 minutes and control responses were recovered about 60 minutes after injection. No comparable effect was observed on glutamate-induced excitation in cells tested alternatively with both transmitters (Figure 5.4). Similar enhancement of ACh effects have subsequently been seen in the *in vitro* hippocampal slice preparation (27), suggesting that this effect is in no way attributable to anesthetic interactions.

In the *in vivo* studies, systemic ethanol also significantly increased the amplitude and duration of inhibitory responses to iontophoretically applied somatostatin-14 (SS-14). This enhancement was also evident within 10 to 15 minutes after ethanol injection, and recovered at 60 to 80 minutes. Ethanol had no statistically significant effect on inhibitory responses to serotonin or adrenaline.

Because of reports that GABA effects are enhanced by very low doses of ethanol (28–30), we also examined hippocampal GABA actions in some detail after ethanol. Although a small (<25%) but consistent potentiation of inhibitory responses to GABA could be observed (26), these potentiations did not recover even 3 hours after ethanol administration. These and other control experiments (26) suggest that the apparent potentiation of GABA was most likely an artifact of the repetitive iontophoretic application under these experimental conditions, rather than a true

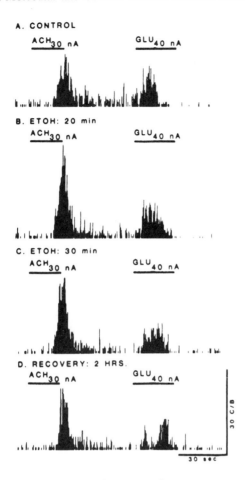

FIGURE 5.4. Ethanol selectively enhances excitatory responses to acetylcholine. Peri–drug-interval histograms, all composed of two sweeps of two drug pulses each. *A*. Control reponses to brief iontophoretic pulses of acetylcholine (ACH) and glutamate (GLU). The subscripts (30 and 40 nA, respectively) indicate the current used to eject the drug; the bar indicates the period of application. Acetylcholine causes a 763% increase in firing rate over baseline; glutamate, an increase of 800%. *B*. Twenty minutes after intraperitoneal ethanol (1.5 g/kg). ACh causes a 1,044% increase in firing above baseline (ie, a 37% larger response than the control), whereas responses to glutamate are not significantly different (836%, or only 4% larger than the control response). *C*. Thirty minutes after ethanol, responses to ACh average 13% larger than control (863% increase above baseline), whereas those of glutamate are 17% smaller than control (662% above baseline). *D*. Recovery from the effects of ethanol is complete after 2 hours. ACh responses are 8% smaller than control (702% above baseline), whereas those of glutamate are 27% smaller (582%). The effect of ethanol on ACh excitations was statistically significant. (matched-pairs sign test, $p < 0.05$) (Calibration: 30 seconds, 30 counts per bin). From Mancillas et al (26). Copyright 1986 by the AAAS.

pharmacological interaction. In contrast, changes in responses to ACh and SS-14 were observed only after ethanol injections and all recovered within 1 to 2 hours.

Subsequently, we have observed that SS-14 itself potentiates responses to ACh in the hippocampus (31). Thus, it is possible that ethanol-induced enhancement of responses to ACh may be secondary to an enhancement of the effects of endogenously related somatostatin, thereby enhancing postsynaptic responses to iontophoretically applied ACh. The ethanol-induced alteration of ACh and SS-14 responses may underlie the enhancement by ethanol of inhibitory and excitatory synaptic transmission previously described in hippocampus (25).

Siggins and colleagues have also examined the effects of ethanol superfusion on the responses of CA1 pyramidal cells to GABA as determined by intracellular recordings *in vitro* and observed that in the dose range of 22–80 mmol/L, ethanol had little effect on the responses to GABA (13). These results thus do not support the conclusion that ethanol enhances GABA-ergic inhibitory postsynaptic potentials (IPSPs). Most recently, Siggins and associates have reported that the potentiation by somatostatin of acetylcholine is mediated through opposing actions on the M-current, although it is not yet clear that ethanol acts at this site (27).

Conclusions on Ethanol Intoxication Effects

Our studies of ethanol intoxication have focused on changes in neuronal properties in four regions of the rodent and primate brain: the cerebellum, the inferior olive, the locus ceruleus, and the hippocampus. In all four regions, systemic ethanol or continuous superfusion *in vitro* produces sensitive effects on selected neuronal properties often at doses below those expected to produce intoxication in humans.

When effects of ethanol are observed in a given brain region, they are consistent and dose-dependent. Based on our overall evaluation to date, we have proposed (3) that the following sequence of events may be critical for intoxication: low doses of ethanol increase variability in responsiveness of locus ceruleus neurons to critical external sensory events, leading to inattention, and decreased arousal. In squirrel monkeys, lesions of the locus ceruleus result in surface potential recording alterations that are similar to those that have been reported in the children of alcoholics, namely a reduced late (P300) potential.

Somewhat higher doses (1 g/kg) of ethanol activate neurons of the inferior olive, possibly indicating the endogenous formation of a serotonin-derived β-carboline–like effect, that depends on the presence of an intact serotonin innervation of the inferior olive. Also at modest doses of ethanol, responses of hippocampal pyramidal neurons to both acetylcholine and somatostatin are enhanced, and the effects of synaptic pathway activation are suppressed. With the exception of the enhanced responsiveness to somatostatin and to acetylcholine during ethanol administration in the hippocampus, no other specific transmitter responses have been observed by us to be influenced by ethanol, including other monoamines or GABA.

However, at least three other neurotransmitter systems have been linked to cellular actions of ethanol by others:

1. The dopaminergic system, where Gessa and colleagues (32–35) have demonstrated not only that low doses of ethanol will excite dopamine-containing neurons of the ventral tegmental area, but also that they will do so only when tested in the unanesthetized state. Furthermore, these investigators have reported that voluntary intake of ethanol in stock populations of rodents will be inhibited by dihydroergotoxine and thioridiazine, actions that may relate to the dopamine receptor interactions of these drugs.

2. The serotonergic system, which has considerable potential involvement beyond our recent observations regarding the necessity of this system for the rate speeding and synchronizing effects of ethanol on neurons of the inferior olivary complex (12). Li and colleagues have established lines of rats bred for the preference of ethanol consumption to moderate intoxicating levels and have shown that among the neurochemical differences between these rats and the control stock lines or lines or alcohol non-preferring behavior is the fact that the brains of ethanol preferring rats are deficient in serotonin (36–39). Interestingly, the examination of the effects of repeated exposure to ethanol suggests that the ''preference'' may in part be based upon a rapid induction of tolerance to the aversive effects of ethanol (38,39). This result might suggest that within this inbred line, even a modest reinforcing action, coupled with reduced potency for actions that may initially be regarded as aversive, could result in a net reinforcing effect of ethanol. Thus it may be considered that rather than suggesting a role for the serotonin system in reinforcement actions per se, the lowered values of 5-HT content might more appropriately be linked to the rapid-tolerance effect with loss of the aversive effects of ethanol.

3. The GABA systems (28–30,40).

Ethanol and GABA-Mediated Behavioral Actions

Results at the behavioral level (30) and more recently at the *in vitro* biochemical level (40–42) have focused attention to ethanol potentiation of GABA-ergic synaptic transmission sites. Koob and his collaborators have found that ethanol and benzodiazepines are synergistic in the anticonflict test mode, and that both drug effects are antagonized by FG 7142 (43) (a carboline ''inverse benzodiazepine agonist'') and by naloxone (44). However, ethanol probably does not release punished responding through direct actions on the primary benzodiazepine receptor. Thus, the drug RO 15-1788, characterized as a benzodiazepine antagonist, does not in fact antagonize the effects of ethanol, although it completely reverses the effects of chlordiazepoxide (43). Nevertheless, as noted above, direct tests of GABA responsiveness (that is, iontophoretic dose-response curves before and after ethanol failed to confirm GABA potentiation in cerebellum (9), as have more recent tests in hippocampus (4,13,26).

Clearly, there are not yet sufficient data to conclude whether GABA-ergic mechanisms per se account for any, many, or all of the intoxicating or reinforcing effects of ethanol. It is possible that the behaviorally arousing effects of GABA-ergic antagonists overcoming ethanol intoxicating could imply a nonspecific summation of more general analeptic actions. It is equally possible that the apparent mimicry of ethanol and GABA effects at both behavioral and multicellular levels may derive from similar but distinct mechanisms. It is noteworthy that our recent intracellular records of CA1 and CA3 pyramidal neurons in the hippocampal slice showed no GABA-like effects (13) (ie, hyperpolarization) and that the GABA-ergic IPSPs evoked by pathway stimulation were most often reduced in size rather than potentiated.

Cellular Actions and Reinforcement

The concern in our present analysis, however, is not with the intoxicating effects of ethanol, but rather with regard to the possibility that one or more of these cellular actions and the underlying, but as yet undocumented, molecular actions on which they are based may represent the basis for the reinforcing effects of ethanol that lead to repeated self-administration of the drug in humans. The same four systems described above—norepinephrine, dopamine, serotonin, and GABA—could also constitute the initiating cellular actions that underlie this effect as well. Wise has argued (45) that there is a single brain reinforcement pathway mechanism that depends upon dopaminergic mechanisms. However, this view appears to be oversimplistic and, as shown by Koob and colleagues (46–48), cannot satisfactorily explain that there are at least two separable anatomic and neurochemical substrates responsible for both cocaine self-administration and heroin self-administration.

Elsewhere, Lewis (49) has provided an overview of the hypotheses that have been invoked in previous analyses to "explain" the reinforcing behavioral effects of ethanol. In his view, only two possibilities have withstood the barrages of contrary and internally inconsistent data that characterizes the ethanol research arena: (a) reinforcement through anxiety-reducing effects of ethanol; and (b) reinforcement through euphorigenic effects of ethanol. On the one hand, the evidence cited above concerning possible GABA-potentiating actions of ethanol has not yet found a basis at the cellular level, while on the other hand the possible dopamine system-stimulating actions of ethanol (32–35) have not been well replicated at the behavioral level in terms of classical reinforcement test systems such as intracranial self-stimulation (49,50). In any case, there is no ready explanation at either the cellular or molecular levels as to how increased dopaminergic synaptic actions can be conceptualized as "mediating" reinforcing actions.

Thus, given the present status of cellular and behavioral data, no single known system precisely matches the profile of actions that could suggest mediation of ethanol reinforcement. Possibly, a combination of anxiolysis (perhaps related to some sites of either GABA or an endogenous benzodiazepine regulation) and euphorigenesis (perhaps mediated by enhanced dopaminergic neuronal activity) could fit this profile more fully.

Proof that an ethanol action may be mediated through a specific chemical form of neurotransmission requires more than testing of exogenous transmitters. A unifying hypothesis of ethanol actions would require that a given system is both necessary and sufficient to explain all relevant actions of ethanol from the most sensitive and earliest effects on neuronal synaptic transmission at discrete ion channel sites through synaptic circuitry, through more global macroelectrode and behavioral actions.

Not only should the ethanol actions be simulated by the appropriate agonist or antagonist of the transmitter hypothesized as critical, but effects on that system must sooner or later be shown to produce similar shifts in the effectiveness of ethanol on membrane processes and behavioral state. For example, our data (18,19) have demonstrated that the synaptic responsiveness of the locus ceruleus (but not its spontaneous activity) certainly ranks among the most sensitive and most rapid actions of ethanol at the whole-animal level. Those data and others obtained elsewhere were used by others to construct the hypothesis that the LC is critical to the changes seen during withdrawal from states of opioid withdrawal or the naloxone-antagonizable suppression of both benzodiazepine- and ethanol-induced increases in punished behavior. The latter hypothesis has been directly tested (51). The data indicate that neither set of psychopharmacological effects (that is, neither naloxone-induced withdrawal symptoms in opiate-dependent rats nor naloxone-sensitive anticonflict effects of ethanol or benzodiazepines) require an intact LC forebrain projection, making this site, despite our obsession with it, an unlikely mediator of these ethanol actions.

Much of the work on attempts to "explain" the actions of ethanol on the brain have historically focused on the ability of ethanol to perturb general membrane functions as measured *in vitro* (52,53). As neuroscientific research proliferates, novel new mechanisms potentially capable of acting as the intermediary of ethanol perturbations will naturally continue to appear. One such recent unexpected intermediate is the evidence suggesting that brain-produced steroids may be selectively and rapidly depleted by low doses of ethanol (54,55). It is further interesting in this regard that the steroids that are produced by the rodent brain are quite similar to synthetic steroids that can be shown to be powerful general anesthetics operating through GABA-like actions (56). Although the brain-produced steroids that have been detected thus far do not share in these actions (Barker, personal communication), it is possible that under the influence of intoxicating doses of ethanol, changes in brain oxidation-reduction reactions may suppress brain steroid synthesis and result in the production of abnormal metabolites of these steroids that in turn could produce some or all of the intoxicating or reinforcing actions.

It is also possible that the corticotropin-releasing factor (CRF) system, known to produce proconflict behavioral effects that are sensitive to ethanol action (42) may underlie the disruption of the locus neurons during intoxication, since this peptide activates the locus (57) but does not facilitate its sensitivity to sensory stimuli. Furthermore, endocrine studies suggest that, in rodents at least, acute ethanol intoxication does release CRF (58).

Although the effects of ethanol on the rodent and primate brain are widespread, there is emerging a specific pattern of ethanol-induced effects that would appear to begin to define the cellular basis for the complex behavioral states termed intoxication, dependence, and tolerance. Recognition of these cellular events and the mechanisms by which ethanol achieves them would in turn seem to be requisite starting points for understanding and perhaps preventing the deleterious dependence that can arise with chronic consumption. Existing data on the biological differences between those humans with high risk for the development of alcoholism and the "control" population (59,60) suggest, on the one hand, that high-risk male alcoholics consistently show reduced responses to ethanol (59) and on the other hand, that this potential genetic disorder may have multiple biological causes that may or may not be attributable to known regulatory effects of specific transmitter-related actions (60).

We look forward to a broadened attack on these targets of ethanol action, within the wider domain of substance abuse research in which the Addiction Research Foundation has been so effective throughout its brief but productive lifetime.

Acknowledgments. The author thanks Nancy Callahan for manuscript typing. This research was supported by USPHS grants from NIAAA (AA-06420, AA-07456) and NIDA (DA-03665).

References

1. American Psychiatric Association (1987). *Alcohol and Health: Sixth Report to Congress.* DHHS Publication 87-1519, US Government Printing Office, Washington, DC, pp 1–147.
2. Blois, MS (1988). Medicine and the nature of vertical reasoning. *N Engl J Med* 318:847–851.
3. Bloom FE (1988). The emerging pharmacology of ethanol *Br J Psychopharmacol* in press.
4. Siggins GR, Bloom FE, French ED, Madamba SF, Mancillas J, Pittman QJ, Rogers J (1987). Electrophysiology of ethanol on central neurons. *Ann NY Acad Sci* 492:350–366.
5. Bloom FE, Siggins GR (1987). Electrophysiological action of ethanol at the cellular level. *Alcohol* 4:331–337.
6. Bloom FE (1975). Conference Summation, in *The Opiate Narcotics,* The International Narcotic Research Club Conference, May 21–24, 1975. Pergamon, New York, pp 251–259.
7. Siggins GR, French E (1979). Central neurons are depressed by iontophoretic and micropressure applications of ethanol and tetrahydropapaveroline. *Drug Alc Depend* 4:239–243.
8. Rogers J, Siggins JR, Schulman JR, Bloom FE (1980). Physiological correlates of ethanol intoxication, tolerance, and dependence in rat cerebellar Purkinje cells. *Brain Res* 196:183–198.
9. Bloom FE, Siggins GR, Foote SL, Gruol D, Aston-Jones G, Rogers J, Pittman Q, Staunton D (1984). Noradrenergic involvement in the cellular actions of ethanol in E Usdin, ed. *Catecholamines, neuropharmacology and central nervous system.* Alan R Liss, New York, pp 159–167.
10. Sinclair JG, Lo GF (1981). The effects of ethanol on cerebellar Purkinje cell discharge pattern and inhibition evoked by local surface stimulation. *Brain Res* 204:465–471.
11. Sinclair JG, Lo GF, Tiem AF (1980). The effects of ethanol on cerebellar Purkinje cells in naive and alcohol-dependent rats. *Can J Physiol Pharmacol* 58:429–432.
12. Rogers J, Madamba SG, Staunton DA, Siggins GR (1986). Ethanol increases single unit activity in the inferior olivary nucleus. *Brain Res* 385:253–262.
13. Siggins GR, Pittman QJ, French ED (1987b). Effects of ethanol on CA1 and CA3 pyramidal cells in the hippocampal slice preparation: An intracellular study. *Brain Res* 414:22–34.
14. Steinbusch HWM (1984). Serotonin-immunoreactive neurons and their projections in the CNS. In A Björklund, T Hökfelt, MJ Kuhar, eds. *Handbook of Chemical Neuroanatomy,* vol 3, *Classical Transmitters and Transmitter Receptors in the CNS, p 2,* Elsevier, New York, pp 68–125.
15. Madamba S, Siggins GR, Battenberg E, Bloom FE (1987). Depletion of brainstem 5-hydroxytryptamine (5-HT) suppresses the excitatory effect of systemic ethanol on inferior olivary neurons (ION). *Soc Neurosci Abstr* 13:501.
16. Daly J, Fuxe K, Jonsson G (1974). 5,7-Dihydroxytryptamine as a tool for the morphological and functional analysis of central 5-hydroxytryptamine neurons. *Res Commun Chem Pathol Pharmacol* 7:175–187.

17. Aston-Jones G, Foote SL, Bloom FE (1982). Low doses of ethanol disrupt sensory responses of brain noradrenergic neurones. *Nature (London)* 296:857–860.
18. Aston-Jones G, Bloom FE (1981). Activity of norepinephrine-containing locus ceruleus neurons in behaving rats anticipates fluctuations in the sleep-waking cycle. *J Neurosci* 1:887–900.
19. Aston-Jones G, Bloom FE (1981). Norepinephrine-containing locus ceruleus neurons in behaving rats exhibit pronounced response to non-noxious environmental stimuli. *J Neurosci* 1:876–886.
20. Foote S, Aston-Jones G, Bloom FE (1980). Impulse activity of locus ceruleus neurons in awake rats and monkeys is a function of sensory stimulation and arousal. *Proc Nat Acad Sci USA* 77:3033–3037.
21. Foote SL, Bloom FE, Aston-Jones G (1983). Nucleus locus ceruleus: new evidence of anatomical and physiological specificity. *Physiol Rev* 63:844–914.
22. Robbins TW, Everitt BJ, Cole BJ (1985). Functional hypotheses of the coeruleocortical noradrenergic projection: a review of recent experimentation and theory. *Physiol Psychol* 13:127–150.
23. Bloom FE (1988). Neurotransmitters: past, present, and future directions. *FASEB* 2:32–41.
24. Pineda J, Foote SL, Neville H (1987). Effects of noradrenergic locus ceruleus lesions on squirrel monkey event-related potentials. *Electroenceph Clin Neurophysiol* 67:77–90.
25. Newlin SA, Mancillas-Trevino J, Bloom FE (1981). Ethanol causes increase in excitation and inhibition in area CA3 of the dorsal hippocampus. *Brain Res* 209:113–128.
26. Mancillas J, Siggins GR, Bloom FE (1986). Systemic ethanol: Selective enhancement of responses to acetylcholine and somatostatin in the rat hippocampus. *Science* 231:161–163.
27. Moore SD, Madamba SG, Joels M, Siggins GR (1988). Somatostatin augments the M-current in hippocampal neurons. *Science* 239:278–280.
28. Nestoros JN (1980). Ethanol specifically potentiates GABA-mediated neurotransmission in feline cerebral cortex. *Science* 209:708–710.
29. Ticku MK, Burch T (1980). Alterations in GABA receptor sensitivity following acute and chronic ethanol treatments. *J Neurochem* 34:417–423.
30. Ticku MK, Burch TP, Davis WC (1983). The interactions of ethanol with the benzodiazepine GABA receptor ionophore complex. *Pharmacol Biochem Behav* 18(Supp):15–18.
31. Mancillas J, Siggins GR, Bloom FE (1986). Somatostatin selectively enhances acetylcholine-induced excitations in rat hippocampus and cortex. *Proc Natl Acad Sci USA* 83:7518–7521.
32. Fadda F, Franch F, Mosca E, Meloni R, Gessa GL (1987). Inhibition of voluntary ethanol intake in rats by a combination of dihydroergotoxine and thioridazine. *Alc Drug Res* 7(4):285–290.
33. Fadda F, Mosca E, Meloni R, Gessa GL (1985–86). Ethanol-stress interaction on dopamine metabolism in the medical prefrontal cortex. *Alc Drug Res* 6(6):449–454.
34. Mereu G, Gessa GL (1985). Low doses of ethanol inhibit the firing of neurons in the substantia nigra, pars reticulata: A GABAergic effect? *Brain Res* 360(1–2):325–330.

35. Gessa GL, Muntoni F, Collu M, Vargiu L, Mereu G (1985). Low doses of ethanol activate dopaminergic neurons in the ventral tegmental area. *Brain Res* 348(1):201–203.
36. Waller MB, Murphy JM, McBride WJ, Lumeng L, Li T-K (1986). Effect of low dose ethanol on spontaneous motor activity in alcohol-preferring and -nonpreferring lines of rats. *Pharmacol Biochem Behav* 24:617–623.
37. Murphy JM, McBride WJ, Lumeng L, Li T-K (1987). Contents of mono-amines in forebrain regions of alcohol-preferring (P) and -nonpreferring (NP) lines of rats. *Pharmacol Biochem Behav* 26:389–392.
38. Gatton GJ, Murphy JM, Waller MB, McBride WJ, Lumeng L, Li T-K (1987). Chronic ethanol tolerance through free-choice drinking in the P line of alcohol-preferring rats. *Pharmacol Biochem Behav* 28:111–115.
39. Gatton GJ, Murphy JM, Waller MB, McBride WJ, Lumeng L, Li T-K (1987). Persistence of tolerance to a single dose of ethanol in the selectively-bred alcohol-preferring P rat. *Pharmacol Biochem Behav* 28:105–110.
40. Kulonen E (1983). Ethanol and GABA. *Med Biol* 61:147–167.
41. Suzdak PD, Glowa, JR, Crawley JN, Schwartz RD, Skolnick P, Paul SM (1986). A benzodiazepine that antagonizes alcohol actions selectively. *Science* 234:1243–1247.
42. Thatcher-Britton K, Ehlers CL, Koob GF (1988). Is ethanol antagonist RO15-4513 selective for ethanol? *Science* 238:648–649.
43. Koob GF, Braestrup C, Thatcher-Britton K (1986). The effects of FG 7142 and RO15-1788 on the release of punished responding produced by chlordiazepox-ide and ethanol in the rat. *Psychopharmacology* 90:173–178.
44. Koob GF, Strecker RE, Bloome FE (1980). Effects of naloxone on the anticonflict properties of alcohol and chlordiazepoxide. *Substance and Alcohol Actions/Misues* 1:447–457.
45. Wise RA (1987). The role of reward pathways in the development of drug dependence. *Pharmacol Ther* 35(1–2):227–263.
46. Pettit HO, Ettenber A, Bloom FE, Koob GF (1984). Destruction of dopamine in the nucleus accumbens selectively attenuates cocaine but not heroin self-administration in rats. *Psychopharmacologia (Berlin)* 84(2):167–173.
47. Koob GF, Pettit HO, Ettenberg A, Bloom FE (1984). Effects of opiate antagonists and their quaternary derivatives on heroin self-administration in the rat. *J Pharmacol Exp Ther* 229(2):481–468.
48. Ettenberg A, Pettit HO, Bloom FE, Koob GF (1982). Heroin and cocaine intravenous self-administration in rats: mediation by separate neural systems. *Psychopharmacologia (Berlin)* 78(3):204–209.
49. Lewis M (1988). Mechanisms of alcohol reinforcement. In *NIAAA Neuro-science Advisory Board Report,* in press.
50. Arregui Aguirre A, Claro Izaguirre F, Goni Garrido MJ, Zarate Oleaga JA, Morgado Bernal I (1987). Effects of acute nicotine and ethanol on medial prefrontal cortex self-stimulation. *Pharmacol Biochem Behav* 27(1):15–20.
51. Koob GF, Thatcher-Britton K, Britton DR, Roberts DCS, Bloom FE (1984). Destruction of the locus ceruleus or the dorsal NE bundle does not alter the release of punished responding by ethanol and chlordiazepoxide. *Physiol Behav* 33:479–485.
52. Goldstein DB (1987). Ethanol-induced adaptation in biological membranes. *Ann NY Acad Sci* 492:103–111.

53. Taraschi TF, Ellingson JS, Rubin E (1987). Membrane structual alterations caused by chronic ethanol consumption: the molecular basis of membrane tolerance. *Ann NY Acad Sci* 492;171–180.
54. Corpechot C, Shoemaker WJ, Bloom FE, Baulieu EE (1983). Endogenous brain steroids: effect of acute ethanol ingestion. *Soc Neurosci Abstr* 13:1237.
55. Vatier OC, Bloom FE (1988). Effect of ethanol on 3 Δ-OH- Δ5 steroid concentration in the rat brain. *Res Soc Alc Abstr* 12:316 (abstract 73).
56. Harrison NL, Vicini S, Barker JL (1987). A steroid anesthetic prolongs inhibitory post-synaptic currents in cultured rat hippocampal neurons. *J Neurosci* 7:604–609.
57. Valentino RJ, Foote SL (1987). Corticotropin-releasing factor disrupts sensory responses of brain noradrenergic neurons. *Neuroendocrinology* 45: 28–36.
58. Rivier C, Rivier J, Vale W (1986). Stress-induced inhibition of reproductive functions: role of endogenous corticotropin-releasing factor. *Science* 231: 607–609.
59. Schuckit MA, Goodwin DA, Winokur GA (1972). A study of alcoholism in half siblings. *Am J Psychiatry* 128:1132.
60. Cloninger CR (1987). Neurogenetic adaptive mechanisms in alcoholism. *Science* 236:410–416.

CHAPTER 6

Presynaptic Inhibition, Presynaptic Facilitation, and the Molecular Logic of Second-Messenger Systems

Andrea Volterra, Steven A. Siegelbaum,
J. David Sweatt, and Eric R. Kandel

Introduction: Mediating and Modulating Synaptic Actions

A striking feature of the organization of the brain is that some synaptic potentials—the signals whereby one cell communicates with another—are fast, lasting only milliseconds, whereas others are slow, lasting many seconds or even many minutes. One of the insights of the last several years is the realization that the two types of synaptic interactions involve two different molecular mechanisms, which result in two different behavioral consequences and are produced by proteins that derive from two distinct gene families (Figure 6.1).

In both types of synaptic actions the receptor acted on by the transmitter has a double function: a recognition function at its receptor site and an effector function at its ion channel. Thus the receptor recognizes the transmitter and instructs the channel to open or close. As shown in Figure 6.1, the channel conducts ions only when it is open (1). In fast synaptic actions, such as those involving the nicotinic acetylcholine (ACh) channels at the neuromuscular junction and the channels regulated in the central nervous system by glutamate, glycine, and γ-aminobutyric acid (GABA) the recognition function (receptor) and the effector function (channel) are carried out by different domains of a common multiple subunit protein (Figure 6.1A). By contrast, slow synaptic actions involve separate proteins for recognition and effector function; the proteins are often at some distance from one another. Remote receptors characterized to date typically consist of a single subunit with seven transmembrane-spanning regions. They communicate with their channels by means of membrane transduction systems such as the proteins that bind guanosine 5'-triphosphate (GTP) and diffusible internal second-messenger systems such as cyclic adenosine monophosphate (cAMP) and the cAMP-dependent protein kinase (Figure 6.1B).

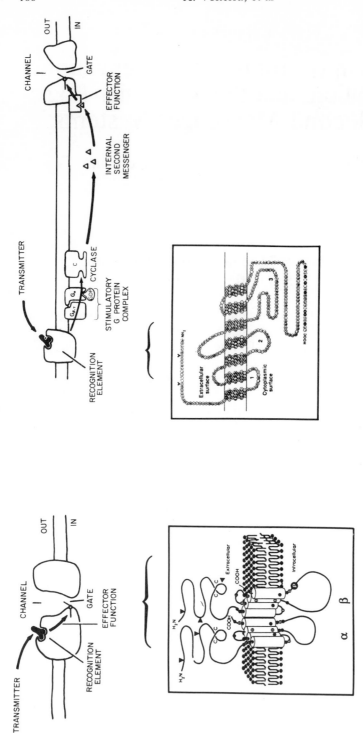

FIGURE 6.1. Schematic diagram illustrating differences between major classes of chemical transmitter actions. A. In mediating synaptic actions, the receptor is an intrinsic part of the transmitter-activated ion channel. These receptors, carrying both recognition and effector function, are typically multisubunit proteins. B. In modulating synaptic actions the receptor is remote from the channel, and coupling depends on a transducing GTP-binding protein and the generation of an intracellular messenger. These receptors are typically single-subunit proteins with several membrane-spanning regions. Adapted from Hille (1).

Slow synaptic actions produced by remote receptors and second messengers have generated much interest because they fulfill quite different functions from the common fast synaptic actions. Whereas the fast synaptic actions produced by the directly acting receptors are utilized by the basic neural circuitry that *mediate* behavior, second messengers produce slow synaptic actions that tend to *modulate* behavior by altering the excitability of neurons and the strength of the synaptic connections of the basic neural circuitry. Specifically, modulatory synaptic pathways can serve as reinforcing stimuli in learning.

The finding that the receptor for the action of some transmitters modulates the channel by means of an internal second messenger opens up the possibility for either synergistic or antagonistic interactions of different transmitters to act on a common channel function. For example, a small family of transmitters, each acting through its own independent remote receptors, may act synergistically to instruct the same channel by means of the same internal second messengers. Alternatively, the receptors could act on the channel antagonistically by means of different internal messengers (Figure 6.2).

We have encountered both of these situations in the studies of the gill withdrawal reflex of *Aplysia californica*. Strong stimuli to the tail of the animal serve as reinforcing stimuli for sensitization and classical conditioning of the reflex. These stimuli activate modulatory neurons that use the transmitter serotonin or the peptides SCP_A and SCP_B. The strong tail stimulus and the transmitter produce presynaptic facilitation at sensorimotor synapses by modulating a specific K^+ channel of the sensory neurons (the S channel) by means of a common second-messenger system, cAMP (2). By contrast, weaker stimuli to the tail that produce inhibition of the reflex activate modulatory neurons that utilize dopamine and the peptide FMRFamide. These weak stimuli and the transmitter systems activate the same S channel in the sensory neurons but now in the opposite way, to produce inhibition acting through the lipoxygenase metabolites of arachidonic acid. Dopamine, binding to a D_2-like receptor, and FMRFamide, have similar actions. We focus here on FMRFamide.

FMRFamide is of further interest, because it resembles the carboxy terminus of the met-enkephalin–related peptide Tyr-Gly-Gly-*Phe-Met-Arg-Phe* (Figure 6.3A). Moreover, Richard Scheller and his colleagues (3) have studied the organization of the FMRFamide precursor polypeptide and have found important similarities with preproenkephalin, one of which is that multiple basic peptide units are interspersed with variable acidic spacers (Figure 6.3B) (4,5). The FMRFamide gene in *Aplysia* encodes at least 19 individual FMRFamide sequences and a single FLRFamide sequence, and gives rise to multiple polyadenylated ribonucleic acids (RNAs). Finally, this structural similarity between FMRFamide and the enkephalin peptides is preserved functionally. Just as enkephalins can produce presynaptic inhibition of nociceptive sensory

A   **SYNAPTIC MODULATION**

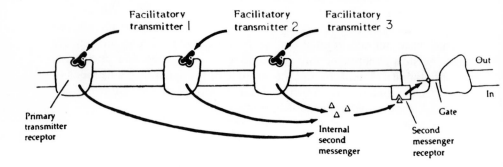

B   **ANTAGONISTIC MODULATION**

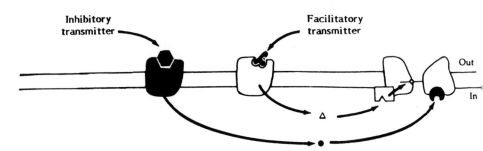

FIGURE 6.2. Possible interactions of modulatory transmitters. *A.* A channel may be linked to several distinct transmitter receptors through a common intracellular messenger. *B.* Different transmitters may produce antagonistic effects on a single ion channel by activating separate second-messenger systems.

neurons in vertebrates, FMRFamide produces presynaptic inhibition of sensory neurons in *Aplysia*.

Indeed, the action of FMRFamide and FMRFamidergic inhibitory interneurons is a mirror image of that of the facilitatory systems. As is the case for the facilitatory neurons, the inhibitory systems synapse onto the sensory neuron's cell body and presynaptic terminals (Figure 6.4). Moreover, we have reason to believe that the K^+ channels, modulated by serotonin and FMRFamide, exist not only in the cell body but also on the terminals, where their modulation plays a role in controlling synaptic strength (6). Thus not only shall we be examining the logic whereby these two transmitters interact within the cell to regulate channel function, acting through two different second messengers, but, in a larger sense, we

FMRFAMIDE   <u>PHE</u> <u>MET</u> <u>ARG</u> <u>PHE</u> <u>NH</u>₂

ENKEPHALIN   <u>TYR</u> <u>GLY</u> <u>GLY</u> <u>PHE</u> <u>MET</u> <u>ARG</u> <u>PHE</u>
RELATED
PEPTIDE

A

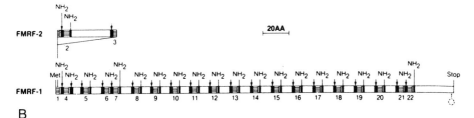

B

FIGURE 6.3. Comparison of sequence and precursor organization between the molluscan neuropeptide FMRFamide and the vertebrate enkephalin peptides. *A.* Sequence homology between FMRFamide and met-enkephalin Arg-Phe, a met-enkephalin–related peptide. *B.* Schematic representation of the precursor polypeptide encoded by *Aplysia* cDNA clones FMRF-1 and FMRF-2. Horizontal lines indicate FMRF amino acid residues, arrows indicate cleavage sites at dibasic residues, lines indicate cleavage sites at single basic residues, and an NH₂ indicates potential amidation sites. The dotted circle indicates a potential glycosylation site at the carboxy terminus of the precursor. The upper schematic represents a region found in clone FMRF-2 but no in FMRF-1. From Schaefer et al (3), copyright © 1985, Cell Press.

also shall be examining how that interaction contributes to the up-and-down regulation of transmitter release. Thus, our data show that the anatomical pathways of the neuronal modulatory circuits are represented at the molecular level within individual nerve cells by the specific molecular circuitry of the second-messenger pathway.

Two features make this interaction of further interest. First, each component is behaviorally relevant. Thus the facilitatory component activated by reinforcing stimuli is important for sensitization and classical conditioning, whereas the inhibitory component is important for behavioral inhibition. Second, the two actions are not symmetrical. The modulatory effects of inhibition are more transient than those of facilitation, but, when present, this transient inhibition can fully override the facilitation.

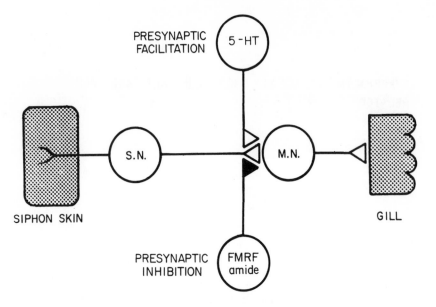

FIGURE 6.4. Circuit diagram for two types of synaptic modulation. In presynaptic facilitation, serotonergic interneurons synapse onto sensory neuron (S.N.) terminals and produce an increase in transmitter release from the sensory neurons onto the follower motor neurons (M.N.). A second class of modulatory interneurons may release FMRFamide and inhibit transmitter release from the sensory neurons.

Presynaptic Facilitation

A strong electrical tail stimulus, presented alone, produces behavioral sensitization of the siphon and gill withdrawal reflex. When it is paired with a stimulus to the siphon, the pairing of the siphon, or conditioned stimulus (CS), with the tail, or unconditioned stimulus (US), leads to classical conditioning.

Both sensitization and classical conditioning lead to an increase in the synaptic strength at the connection between the sensory neuron and the motor neuron mediating the withdrawal reflex. In both cases, tail stimuli activate the facilitatory system. Although we do not know all of the elements of the facilitatory system or all the transmitters these elements use, we have identified two groups of facilitating cells and have reason to believe there is a third. Each of these three groups uses a different transmitter:

1. Serotonin, released by the LC_B and RC_v cells.
2. An as-yet-unidentified transmitter that may be related to serotonin, released by the L29 cells.
3. Two small interrelated peptides, SCP_A and SCP_B.

Processes containing these peptides come in close apposition to those of the sensory neuron in the neuropile, but their cell bodies have not yet been identified.

During classical conditioning, the pairing of the CS and US leads to amplification of presynaptic facilitation. When the CS, which excites the siphon sensory neurons, is paired with the US, which produces the facilitatory input, the response of sensory neurons to the facilitatory input is enhanced. We have called this enhancement *activity-dependent enhancement* of presynaptic facilitation. Because the siphon sensory neurons are responsible for the afferent input to the reflex from the conditioned stimulus, this associative presynaptic facilitation of their synaptic connections is an important contributor to the associative changes produced by conditioning in this system. Similar activity-dependent synaptic facilitation was found by Walters and Byrne in the pleural sensory neurons that innervate the tail in *Aplysia*. Both studies illustrate that an associative interaction produced by learning can occur with an individual neuron.

Conventional presynaptic facilitation, which occurs when the facilitatory input arrives in the absence of paired-spike activity and contributes to sensitization of the withdrawal reflex, is mediated by increased cAMP levels and cAMP-dependent protein phosphorylation in the sensory neurons. Activity-dependent enhancement of presynaptic facilitation augments several presynaptic actions produced during conventional presynaptic facilitation (see below). In both the siphon sensory neurons and in closely related mechanosensory neurons in the pleural ganglion of *Aplysia* (studied by Walters and Byrne), the rise in cAMP produced by brief applications of the facilitatory transmitter serotonin is greater if the cells are depolarized to fire action potentials just before they are exposed to transmitter.

The siphon is innervated by a cluster of about 24 sensory cells. These neurons make excitatory monosynaptic connections with interneurons and motor neurons that produce the withdrawal reflex. Here, we will focus exclusively on the monosynaptic portion of the reflex circuit consisting of the sensory neuron, the motor neuron, and their connections. Other changes also occur at other loci within the neural circuit, but we will not consider these changes.

Based on voltage clamp and biochemical studies of the sensory neuron, both in the intact ganglion and in dissociated cell culture, we have outlined a molecular model for presynaptic facilitation; for an earlier view, see Kandel and Schwartz (7). According to this view, serotonin (as well as the other facilitating transmitters), released by the facilitating neurons, activates a transmitter-sensitive adenylate cyclase in the membrane of the sensory neuron, including its presynaptic terminal, that increases the level of intracellular cAMP. The cAMP then activates a protein kinase that phosphorylates a number of substrate proteins including a K^+-channel protein or a protein associated with it (8,9). This phosphorylation causes closure of the K^+ channels, reducing one of the K^+ conductances that normally repolarize the action potential. Reduction of this conductance produces three consequences: It depolarizes the cell; it increases the excitability of the neuron and prolongs the action potential so as to allow more Ca^{++} flow into the terminals; finally, it contributes to increased release of transmitter (8,10–14). Biochemical evidence for the role of cAMP in facilitation is consistent with the physiological effect of serotonin and cAMP on transmitter release. In physiological experiments we found that 5-HT and intracellular injection of cAMP or the cAMP-dependent protein kinase simulate presynaptic facilitation (Figure 6.5). Independent of K-channel closure, serotonin also alters the handling of Ca^{++} within the sensory neurons, thereby leading to a rise in free intracellular Ca^{++} (15,16). This rise in free Ca^{++} may be important for the mobilization of transmitter in the face of continued transmitter release (13,14). We here focus on only one of the effects of 5-HT and cAMP: their action on the K^+ channel.

Serotonin Decreases the Number of Open K^+ Channels

What are the properties of the K^+ channel modulated by 5-HT? Single-channel recordings from membranes of the sensory neurons revealed that the serotonin-sensitive K^+ channel has novel properties (17). The channel is active at the resting potential. Its gating is not affected by the activity of intracellular calcium ions and shows only a moderate dependence on membrane potential (Figure 6.6).

This initial analysis allowed us to address the next question: How does 5-HT modulate this channel? The total current flow (I) through populations of an ion channel is given by $I = N \times p \times i$. Does 5-HT affect the number of (N) of functional channels in the patch? The probability (p) of channel opening? Or the elementary conductance (i) of the channel (Figure 6.7)?

We have found that serotonin appears to reduce the *number* of functional channels in a patch of membrane and it does so in an all-or-nothing manner (Figure 6.8). Channels that still open in the presence of 5-HT appear to open and close normally, whereas channels once closed by 5-HT remain closed. The modulatory action of serotonin does not involve either a change in the channel's ionic specificity or detectable changes in single-channel conductance over the lifetime of the channel in the open state. Rather, serotonin greatly increases the lifetime of the channel in a close state. This effect may simply represent the modification of the normal channel-gating process whereby one of the normal rate constants of channel opening is dramatically decreased. Alternatively, serotonin may induce new closed states of the channel (perhaps corresponding to the channel in a phosphorylated form) in which the channel is not available to the normal gating process.

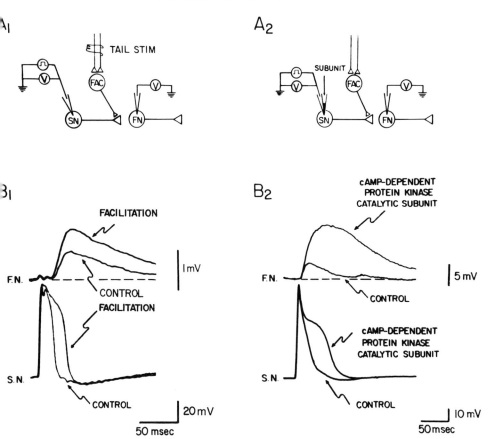

FIGURE 6.5. The effects of presynaptic facilitation on duration of the action potential and synaptic strength are replicated by injecting the cAMP-dependent protein kinase into the sensory neuron. A_1. Experimental arrangement used to elicit ordinary presynaptic facilitation. An electrode is used to stimulate a sensory neuron intracellularly while a shock is delivered to the animal's tail, exciting a facilitatory interneuron that also synapses on the sensory neuron. The response is recorded in a follower (motor) neuron (F.N). A_2. Experimental arrangement for mimicking the effect of presynaptic facilitation by stimulating the sensory neuron intracellularly, as in A_1, but replacing the tail shock with an intracellular injection of the catalytic subunit of the protein kinase directly into the sensory neuron. B_1. The presynaptic facilitation produced by activating a single facilitatory interneuron (as in A_1) is compared with the response produced in a follower neuron by simple stimulation of a sensory neuron (control). B_2. The action potential that results when the catalytic subunit of the protein kinase is injected into the sensory neuron very closely resembles that produced by ordinary presynpatic facilitation. In both cases, the action potential is broadened, leading to an enhancement of transmitter release and a heightened response in the follower neuron. From Castellucci et al (8).

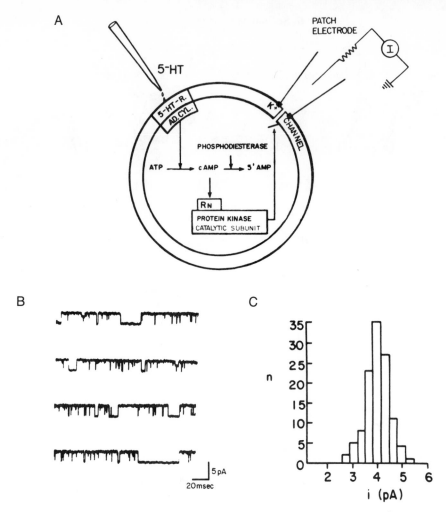

FIGURE 6.6 Patch clamp recording of a single S channel current. *A*. Schematic illustration of the experimental recording protocol and the model from cAMP-dependent action of 5-HT. A high-resistance (gigaohms) seal is obtained between the extracellular patch electrode and the cell membrane to record single-channel currents in the small patch of membrane under the electrode. The recording configuration shown is the cell-attached mode. Serotonin is applied to the cell outside the membrane patch but may still alter channel activity in the patch via the cAMP cascade. The substrate protein for the kinase may or may not be the S channel itself. *B*. Serotonin-sensitive K^+ channel. Single-channel current records from mechanoreceptor sensory neurons (LE cluster) in the abdominal ganglion of *Aplysia californica*. Both the bath and recording pipette contain artificial seawater. Channel openings appear as step increases outward current (outward current plotted in upward direction). The current fluctuates between two levels corresponding to the fully closed and fully open channel. The channel shows both brief closures (downward flickers) and long closures but is in the open configuration for most of the time. Addition of 10 μmol/L serotonin in the bath caused this channel to close (see Figure 6.8). *C*. Histogram of single-channel current amplitudes measured at +11 mV. Reprinted by permission from *Nature* (1982); 299:413–417. Copyright © 1982 Macmillan Magazines Ltd.

CONTROL   + 5 - H T

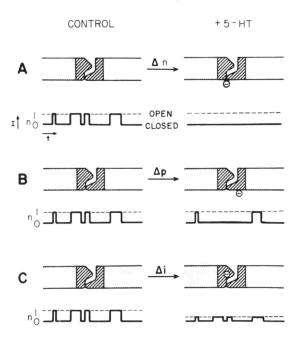

FIGURE 6.7. Possible modes of modulatory transmitter action on single-channel currents. The drawings depict channels as integral membrane proteins with an aqueous pore for ion permeation and a gate for controlling channel opening and closing. Idealized current records show channel openings as an upward current deflection. Transmitter could, in principle, lead to a decrease in the average current carried by a population of such channels by modulating (A) number N of functional channels, (B) the probability of p of channel opening, or (C) the amplitude i of the single-channel current, giving rise to different changes in single-channel function. Modified from Siegelbaum and Tsien (18).

Cyclic Amp and the Cyclic Amp-Dependent Protein Kinase Cause Channel Closure Similar to That Produced by Serotonin

The patch pipette in the cell-attached mode forms a very stable, high-resistance seal with the membrane that is thought to prevent diffusion of transmitters or other ligands from outside to inside the pipette. As a result, in the ACh-activated channels of muscle, the transmitter has to be introduced in the patch pipette to affect the channels under the pipette. By contrast, serotonin decreased the K^+ channel opening in the sensory cell membrane patch when applied to the bathing solution outside the pipette (Figure 6.6). This finding is consistent with the notion that the modulation of the K^+ channel is mediated by a second messenger that connects the 5-HT receptor to the S channel under the pipette by diffusion within the cell. To test this idea directly, we injected the cell with cAMP, the second messenger thought to modulate the serotonin-sensitive K^+

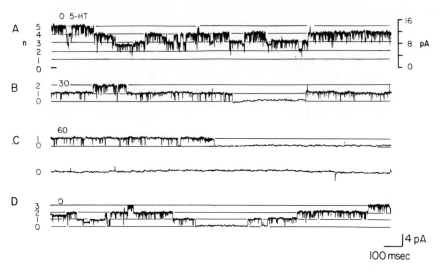

FIGURE 6.8. Action of serotonin (5-HT) on single-channel current. Patch clamp current recorded from mechanoreceptor sensory neurons in the abdominal ganglion of *Aplysia californica*. *A*. Current in the absence of serotonin. Left-hand ordinate shows the number of open channels; right-hand ordinate shows current magnitude. Individual current steps are 2.6 pA. The current record was well fitted by a binomial distribution assuming that five channels are active in the patch and that each channel opens with a probability of 0.84. *B*. Current obtained 2 minutes after addition of 30 μmol/L serotonin to the bath. *C*. Current 1 minute after addition of a further dose of serotonin, raising the total concentration to 60 μmol/L. The two traces are a continuous recording. *D*. Current recorded after washout of serotonin. Reprinted by permission from *Nature* (1982). 299:413–417. Copyright © 1982 Macmillan Magazines Ltd.

current. As with serotonin, intracellular injection of cAMP, by means of current pulses, causes channels to close in an all-or-none manner. In the experiment illustrated by Figure 6.9*A,* three channels are active before the start of the current injection (trace 1). After the onset of the current pulses, these channels drop out, one at a time (trace 2). Similar effects are seen following application of the catalytic subunit of the cAMP-dependent protein kinase to the inside surface of an isolated membrane patch (Figure 6.9*B*). These results suggest that cAMP-dependent protein kinase leads to all-or-none closures of the S channels by acting on a membrane associate substrate protein, either the S channel itself or a regulatory protein that acts on the channel.

Presynaptic Inhibition

How does behavioral inhibition work? Studies by Mackey, Glanzman, Hawkins, and Small suggest that the behavioral inhibition is reflected at the level of the sensory neuron by presynaptic inhibition of transmitter

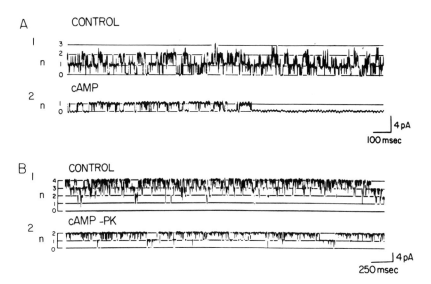

FIGURE 6.9. *A*. Action of cAMP and the catalytic unit of cAMP-protein kinase on single-channel current recorded from sensory neurons in the abdominal ganglion of *Aplysia californica*. A. Trace 1 shows the current in the absence of cAMP. Left-hand ordinate shows the number of open channels. Trace 2 shows the effect of intracellular injection of cAMP on single-channel current. Following establishment of the seal between patch electrode and membrane, the cell was impaled with a microelectrode filled with 1 μmol/L cAMP (Sigma) and cAMP was injected into cells by hyperpolarizing current pulses. Note that only one active channel is open and after a while this last channel is closed. From Siegelbaum et al (17). *B*. Effect of cAMP-kinase on S channels in inside-out membrane patches from sensory neurons. In trace 1, before the addition of the kinase, the patch contained four active channels open for a large fraction of the time. In trace 2, taken 3 minutes after addition of cAMP-PK (0.1 μmol/L final concentration) plus 1 mmol/L Mg-ATP, two channels have closed and the current level fluctuates from zero to two channels open. Reprinted by permission from *Nature* (1985); 313:392–395. Copyright © 1985 Macmillan Magazines Ltd.

release, a mirror image to the process of presynaptic facilitation. However, behavioral inhibition has the added feature that, although it is brief, it is capable of overriding the effects of facilitation. Behavioral inhibition is mediated in part by the peptide FMRFamide. Small, Hawkins, and Kandel have identified an interneuron, located within the left pleural ganglion, that shows FMRFamide immunoreactivity. This interneuron is activated by tail shock and, when stimulated with current pulses, simulates the presynaptic inhibitory action produced by tail shock. Dale and Kandel have found that FMRFamide leads to a decrease in spontaneous transmitter release from the presynaptic terminal of the sensory neuron without affecting the size of the quantal responses. This finding indicates that the sensitivity of receptors of the postsynaptic cell for the transmitter FMRFamide is not affected.

A. Volterra, et al

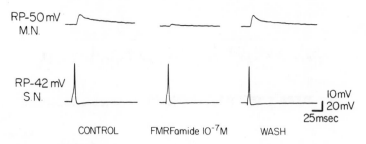

FIGURE 6.10. FMRFamide inhibits synaptic transmission between sensory and motor neurons in culture. Effect on EPSP is shown. Top trace shows fast EPSP in the motor neuron in response to stimulation of the sensory neuron (shown in bottom trace). FMRFamide produces a reversible decrease in the size of the EPSP in the motor neuron.

What are the molecular and ionic mechanisms of presynaptic inhibition (Figure 6.10)? When applied onto a sensory neuron, FMRFamide produces a slow, transient hyperpolarization, an increase in membrane conductance, and a narrowing of the action potential (Figure 6.11A; see also upper traces in Figures 6.20A and B). To produce hyperpolarization and narrowing of the action potential, FMRFamide alters several macroscopic currents. It increases a background K^+ current and decreases a voltage-dependent Ca^{++} current and a Ca^{++}-dependent K^+ current (6,19,20). We have here restricted our patch clamp analysis to the actions on the background K current. Specifically, we have explored whether FMRFamide modulates the same class of K^+ channels closed by 5-HT. If so, which parameter of S channel function is altered? Finally, how do 5-HT and FMRFamide interact in causing channel modulation and what is at the single-channel level the mechanism of the inhibitory override?

FMRFamide Modulates Single S Channels

Single-channel current recordings indicate that the slow hyperpolarization produced by FMRFamide is indeed associated with an increase in the opening of S channels (Figure 6.11).

We have seen above that serotonin decreases the macroscopic S current by causing prolonged all-or-none S-channel closures, resulting in an apparent decrease in the number of functional channels in the membrane. We were therefore interested in knowing: Does FMRFamide increase the mean S-channel current by increasing N, p, or i (Figure 6.12)? We found that FMRFamide produces no marked change in either the single-channel amplitude (i) or in the maximum number of channels that open simultaneously (N_f). A plot of the single-channel-unit current-

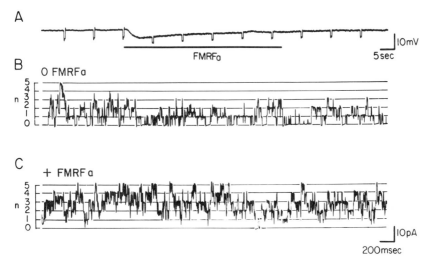

FIGURE 6.11. FMRFamide action on pleural sensory neurons. *A.* FMRFamide produces a slow hyperpolarization of the cell resting potential accompanied by an increase in membrane conductance. The application of 2 μmol/L FMRFamide is indicated by the solid line. Constant-current hyperpolarizing pulses of 0.1 nA were delivered to the cell to monitor membrane conductance. *B, C.* Effect of FMRFamide (2μmol/L on single-channel current. Trace *B* shows channel currents before addition of FMRFamide, and trace *C* shows the increase in channel current approximately 10 minutes after addition of 2 μmol/L FMRFamide to the bath. Approximate patch membrane potential was +20 mV, assuming a resting potential of −60 mV. Reprinted by permission from *Nature* (1987); 325:153–156. Copyright © 1987 Macmillan Magazines Ltd.

voltage relation before and after FMRFamide confirms the lack of change in the elementary current i (Figure 6.13*A*).

A more quantitative test of whether FMRFamide alters N_f or p was obtained from a fit of the binomial distribution to the observed probability distribution that a given number of channels in the patch are open simultaneously. The results show that, whereas FMRFamide produces a clear increase in p, N remains essentially the same (Figures 6.13*B* and *C*).

The most convincing demonstration that FMRFamide acts to increase p rather than N_f was achieved with a patch containing only one active S channel. Figure 6.14 shows a continuous single-channel record on a slow time scale from such a patch. Before application of FMRFamide, the channel in this patch showed occasional brief openings that appear as upward spikes on this slow time scale. However, within 1 minute after application of FMRFamide, there is a marked increase in opening of the one S channel. Inasmuch as we never observed more than a single channel open in the presence of FMRFamide, despite the dramatic rise in channel-open probability, FMRFamide must act to increase p rather than N_f.

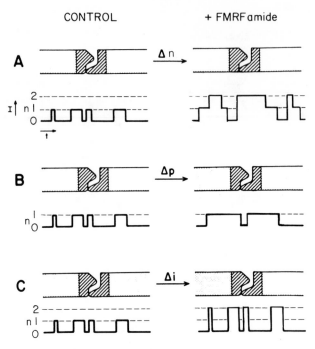

FIGURE 6.12. Possible modes of FMRFamide action at the level of single channel currents. In principle, FMRFamide could lead to an increase in actual K^+ current by (A) increasing the functional number of active channels; (B) increasing the probability of opening a single channel; and (C) increasing single-channel conductance. Reprinted by permission from *Nature* (1987); 325:153–156. Copyright © 1987 Macmillan Magazines Ltd.

FMRFamide Overrides the Action of 5-HT at the Single-Channel Level

The behavioral finding that inhibition can override facilitation and the cellular finding that both act on a common channel raises the question: How do the two modulatory inputs interact in modulating the S channel (Figure 6.15)? We found first that FMRFamide antagonizes and overrides the slow excitatory action of serotonin (or cAMP) at the level of membrane potential. The single-channel basis for this override is shown in Figures 6.16 and 6.17. The patch of membrane illustrated in Figure 6.16 and analyzed in Figure 6.17 initially displayed four active S channels (control). On application of dibutyryl cAMP to the bath, two of the four active channels close (cAMP), leading to a decrease in N_f as described

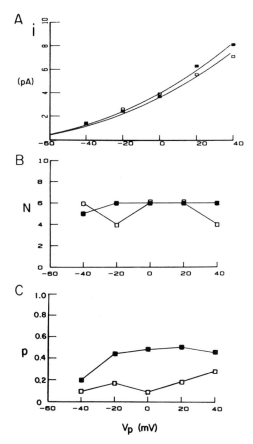

FIGURE 6.13. Analysis of the action of FMRFamide on single-S-channel current. *A.* Relationship between single open channel current i and membrane patch potential V_p before (open squares) and after (filled squares) FMRFamide. Solid line shows least-squares fit, of the Goldman-Hodgkin-Katz constant field current equation, for a pure K current to the data. *B, C.* Maximum likelihood estimates from binomial analysis for N_f and p over a wide range of membrane potentials before (open squares) or after (filled squares) FMRFamide. The open probability of the S channels shows only a moderate dependence on membrane potential in the absence or presence of FMRFamide, with a twofold to threefold increase in p for an 80-mV depolarization. Reprinted by permission from *Nature* (1987); 325:153–156. Copyright © 1987 Macmillan Magazines Ltd.

earlier (Figures 6.16 and 6.17; cAMP). The two remaining active channels appear normal, with no change in single-channel amplitude or open probability. We then applied FMRFamide to the cell, still in the presence of cAMP (Figure 6.16 and 6.17; cAMP-FMRFamide). Now, in addition to the normal increase in open probability, the peptide also produces an increase in the number of functional channels from two up to the original

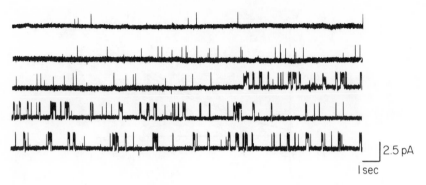

FIGURE 6.14. Effect of FMRFamide on a patch with a single S channel. Consecutive sweeps illustrating transition from low-probability gating to high-probability gating in response to 20 μmol/L FMRFamide. The membrane potential was approximately +20 mV. Records were filtered at 500 Hz. The peptide was applied 20 seconds before the start of the top trace. Reprinted by permission from *Nature* (1987); 325:153–156. Copyright © 1987 Macmillan Magazines Ltd.

level of four (Figure 6.17). This finding is in contrast to the single action FMRFamide to increase p in the absence of cAMP. The ability of FMRFamide to reopen channels closed by cAMP strengthens the argument that the peptide does indeed modulate the same class of S channels closed by cAMP and 5-HT. It also suggests that FMRFamide action does not require a decrease in adenylate cyclase activity.

These results show that the S channel can be modulated in opposite directions during presynaptic facilitation produced by serotonin and during presynaptic inhibition produced by FMRFamide (Figure 6.18). However, the modes of action of these modulatory transmitters differ in fundamental ways. Serotonin causes prolonged channel closures, resulting in a decrease in the number of functional channels (Figure 6.18A); normally, FMRFamide acts to increase channel opening without increasing the number of functional channels (Figure 6.18B). These observations

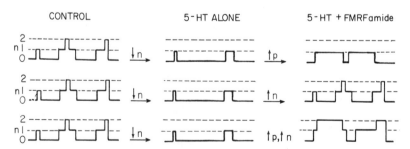

FIGURE 6.15. Diagram of the ways FMRFamide can increase the average currents through the S K$^+$ channels in the presence of 5-HT. See text for explanation.

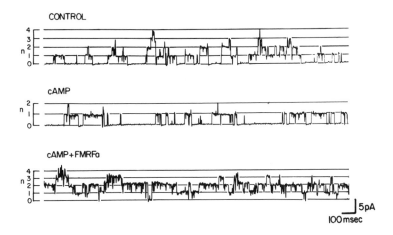

FIGURE 6.16. FMRFamide antagonizes the action of 5-HT and cAMP. On the level of single channels, FMRFamide antagonizes the closure of channels induced by cAMP. Top trace is a current record from patch containing four active S channels before application of cAMP. Middle trace is a current record obtained 10 minutes after addition of 0.1 mmol/L dibutyryl cAMP to bath showing closure of two channels. Closures occurred within 5 minutes after addition of cAMP and persisted in maintained presence of cAMP until addition of FMRFamide. Lower trace is a current record 5 minutes after application of 2 μmol/L FMRFamide (still in presence of cAMP), showing reopening of two channels and increase in open probability. Membrane potential was about 20 mV; current records were filtered at 1 kHz. Reprinted by permission from *Nature* (1987); 325:153–156. Copyright © 1987 Macmillan Magazines Ltd.

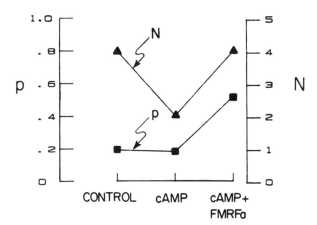

FIGURE 6.17. Results of binomial analysis of several minute-long stretches of data showing maximum-likelihood estimates for N_f (triangles) and p (squares) in control conditions (leftmost points), in presence of cAMP alone (middle points) and in the presence of both cAMP and FMRFamide (rightmost points). Reprinted by permission from *Nature* (1987); 325:153–156. Copyright © 1987 Macmillan Magazines Ltd.

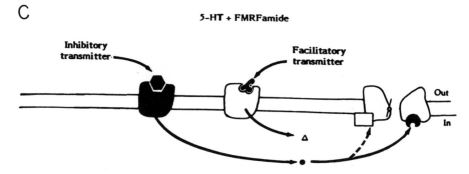

FIGURE 6.18. Summary of modulatory actions on S channel by the presynaptic facilitatory and inhibitory transmitters. *A.* 5-HT, the facilitatory transmitter, leads to S-channel closure via cAMP-dependent phosphorylation. *B.* FMRFamide, the inhibitory transmitter, acts via an unidentified second messenger to increase the probability of an S-channel opening. *C.* FMRFamide is capable of reopening channels closed by 5-HT, suggesting an antagonistic action at either the site on the channel altered with 5-HT or some other step in the phosphorylation-depolarization reaction.

imply that the S channel has two distinct functional sites of modulation that may correspond to separate structural sites on the channel. Nevertheless, the two transmitter effects are not completely independent. In addition to increasing channel-open probability, FMRFamide is able to override the action of 5-HT by reopening channels closed by cAMP (Figure 6.18C). This feature suggests that FMRFamide may have several sites of action. One possibility is that in addition to an action at a site on the channel involved in gating, FMRFamide may also stimulate phosphatase activity to reverse cAMP- and cAMP-dependent protein kinase-induced channel closures.

FMRFamide Also Overrides the Pattern of Substrate Protein Phosphorylation Produced by 5-HT and cAMP

The inhibitory override can be explored at the molecular level. Sweatt and Kandel found that a single pulse of 5-HT or of cAMP to intact sensory neurons activates an identical and specific pattern of phosphorylation as determined by quantitative two-dimensional gels. Serotonin or cAMP increases the level of phosphorylation of 17 substrate proteins. These proteins range in molecular weight from 20,000 to 60,000 and in pI (or isolectric pH) from 4.5 to 7.5 No proteins have their phosphorylation decreased in response to 5-HT or cAMP. The alteration of a relatively large number of proteins suggests that the action of 5-HT is not limited only to the K^+ channel but extends to a wide variety of biochemical processes within the sensory neurons.

Sweatt, Volterra, Siegelbaum, and Kandel have now asked the question: How does FMRFamide act on this set of biochemical processes? They have found that acting alone, FMRFamide *decreases* the basal level of phosphorylation of 10 of the 17 proteins phosphorylated by 5-HT and cAMP. No proteins show an increase in phosphorylation with FMRFamide. When presented together with 5-HT, FMRFamide completely overrides the action of 5-HT or cAMP. Thus, FMRFamide shows, on a molecular level, the inhibitory override evident on both the behavioral and cellular levels.

Additional evidence for the inhibitory override comes from recent studies of Volterra and Siegelbaum, who showed that the modulatory actions of 5-HT and FMRFamide on the S channel are both mediated by GTP-binding proteins (G proteins), even if the two G proteins involved in FMRFamide and 5-HT action are of a different kind. Intracellular injection into the sensory neuron of GTP-gamma-S, a GTP analog capable of activating all G proteins in a nonselective manner, however, results in the mimicking of just the FMRFamide effect. The 5-HT-related effect of GTP-γ-S is unmasked only when the intracellular FMRFamide cascade is pharmacologically blocked (21).

The Receptors for Presynaptic Inhibition and Presynaptic Facilitation Activate Separate Intracellular Second-Messenger Systems

Since application of FMRFamide to the bath is capable of opening channels under the patch pipette that have no direct access to the peptide, the peptide is most probably acting through a second-messenger system. As serotonin closes the S channels through the cAMP pathway, an obvious possibility is that FMRFamide decreases the resting cAMP concentration and thus leads to channel opening. However, biochemical measurements of Ocorr and Byrne (22) show no change in levels of cAMP in sensory neurons in response to FMRFamide. Our single-channel results also do not support a decrease in cAMP as the mode of FMRFamide action, because such an effect would be expected to lead to an increase in the number of functional channels (N_f) in the patch (ie, the converse of the action of 5-HT) rather than to the increase in open probability observed. Thus, FMRFamide uses a second-messenger pathway that does not seem to involve adenylate cyclase modulation. Studies from our laboratory and others seem to rule out the possibility that known second messengers—such as IP3, diacylglycerol, or cGMP—mediate FMRFamide action on the S channel (12,20).

A possible mechanism for generating second-messenger molecules for neuronal signaling is the receptor-mediated release of arachidonic acid from membrane phospholipids. Release of arachidonic acid has been well characterized in nonneural cells, where free arachidonate is rapidly metabolized to eicosanoids, a family of active products that are thought to be both intracellular and intercellular messengers (23). Although the metabolism of arachidonic acid in the brain has been studied for more than 20 years (28,29) the complexity of the mammalian central nervous system has made it difficult to assign specific functions to the eicosanoids. In collaboration with J. H. Schwartz and D. Piomelli, we decided to study the arachidonic acid metabolism in *Aplysia* taking advantage of the simpler nervous system of this marine mollusk, where it is possible to examine identified nerve cells of known behavioral function both in intact ganglia and in dissociated cells in culture. Our results indicate that the inhibitory synaptic actions of FMRFamide are mediated by lipoxygenase metabolites of arachidonic acid (29).

The Eicosanoid Pathways in Aplysia

Schwartz and his colleagues have found that arachidonate is a prominent component of *Aplysia* neural phospholipids (about 10% of total fatty acid content) and can be metabolized in *Aplysia* neurons through both the 12-lipoxygenase and the 5-lipoxygenase pathways, as well as through the cyclo-oxygenase pathway (30). These pathways are drawn in Figure 6.19,

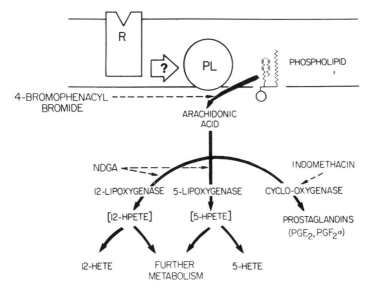

FIGURE 6.19. Pathways of arachidonic acid metabolism in neural tissue of *Aplysia californica*. In mammals, arachidonic acid release is catalyzed by a phospholipase A_2 or by the combined action of a phospholipase C and a diacylglycerol-lipase (PL); see Irvine (38). Both enzymes can be stimulated in a receptor-mediated (R) fashion and are irreversibly inhibited by 4-bromophenacyl bromide; see Blackwell and Flower (32). In *Aplysia*, Piomelli et al (30) have found that esterified arachidonate accounts, on average, for 10% of total fatty acids in neural phospholipids. Free arachidonic acid can be metabolized in *Aplysia* neural tissue through the 12-lipoxygenase, the 5-lipoxygenase, and the cyclo-oxygenase pathways. Two lipoxygenase products, 12-hydroxy eicosatetraenoic acid (12-HETE) and 5-HETE have been identified. These stable end products are not further metabolized and are thought to be derived from the corresponding unstable hydroperoxy acids (HPETE). The lipoxygenase reaction is selectively inhibited by low concentrations of nordihydroguaiaretic acid (NDGA). *Aplysia* neural tissue also has a cyclo-oxygenase activity and forms several prostaglandins, of which PGE_2 and $PGF_{2\alpha}$ have been identified. Prostaglandin formation is inhibited by indomethacin. Reprinted by permission from *Nature* (1987); 328:38–43. Copyright © 1987 Macmillan Magazines Ltd.

which also indicates the sites of action of the various drugs that we used in this study. Two stable lipoxygenase products, the hydroxy acids 12-HETE and 5-HETE, have been identified in neural tissue from *Aplysia* (30). In mammals, these hydroxy acids are formed by enzymatic reduction of the corresponding short-lived hydroperoxides (HPETE) (33). The presence of hydroperoxy acids is only inferred in *Aplysia*, since we have not yet isolated these unstable precursors. Both 12-HPETE and 5-HPETE may be metabolized to products other than the hydroxy acids (23). Finally, the cyclo-oxygenase pathway leads to the synthesis of various prostaglandins which in *Aplysia* nervous tissue include PGE_2 and $PGF_{2\alpha}$ (30).

Arachidonate Mimics FMRFamide

To investigate the possible physiological role of arachidonic acid metabolites, we first applied arachidonate extracellularly by pressure ejection onto the sensory neurons from a large pipette (34). Arachidonic acid

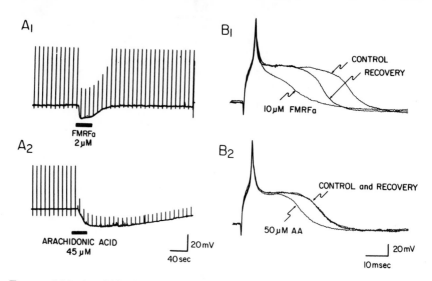

FIGURE 6.20. Arachidonic acid simulates the action of FMRFamide on whole-cell potential responses. *A*. Changes in membrane potential and spike firing of sensory neurons in culture in response to (A_i) FMRFamide (2 μmol/L) or (a_2) arachidonic acid (45 μmol/L). The solid bar indicates period of application. Intracellular records are from the same cell. Initial resting potential was −41 mV in A_1 and −35 mV in A_2. Upward spikes are action potentials elicited once every 10 seconds by brief depolarizing (constant) current stimuli. The smaller spikes reflect action potential inhibition and are the passive depolarizing responses to the current step. The slower time course of the arachidonic-induced hyperpolarization most likely reflects the time required for diffusion (or transport) across the plasma membrane and metabolism *B*. FMRFamide and arachidonate cause a reversible decrease in action potential duration. Action potentials recorded from sensory neuron in an intact abdominal ganglion in presence of 50 mmol/L tetraethylammonium (control). In absence of TEA, decrease in action potential duration is also observed with FMRFamide and arachidonic acid; however, the brief duration of the control action potential makes shortening difficult to measure accurately. Resting potential in B_1 was −43 mV before FMRFamide and −48 mV in presence of peptide. In B_2, resting potential was −43 mV before arachidonate and −44.5 mV in presence of the fatty acid. In the intact ganglia, response to arachidonic acid is somewhat smaller and slower than in culture, probably due to the restricted access and diffusion of the fatty acid. Reprinted by permission from *Nature* (1987); 328:38–43. Copyright © 1987 Macmillan Magazines Ltd.

simulated the macroscopic actions of FMRFamide, producing a slow hyperpolarization of the membrane associated with an increase in membrane conductance (not shown), decreasing the duration of the action potential (Figure 6.20), and inhibiting synaptic transmission between the sensory neuron and motor neuron (Figure 6.21). Eicosa-11-monoenoic acid, a 20-carbon-chain fatty acid with one double bond, which constitutes 4.3% of *Aplysia* neural fatty acids (30) had little effect on resting potentials, action potentials, or synaptic potentials.

The similarity between the physiological effects of FMRFamide and arachidonic acid results from their sharing common ionic mechanisms. Voltage clamp experiments on sensory neurons in culture show that arachidonic acid and FMRFamide produce similar effects on the membrane current-voltage relation (Figure 6.22).

To obtain more direct evidence that FMRFamide and arachidonic acid share a common mode of action, we studied single S-channel currents in cell-attached membrane patches (Figure 6.23). In the experiment shown in Figure 6.23, FMRFamide caused a fivefold to sixfold increase in mean S-channel current over a range of membrane voltages (Figure 6.23B_1) with no significant effect on the single-channel current amplitude(Figure 6.23C_1). Arachidonic acid caused a twofold to fourfold increase in mean channel current (Figure 6.23B_2) with no significant effect on single-channel amplitude (Figure 6.23C_2). Using a binomial analysis, we were able to confirm that the mode of action of arachidonic acid is similar to

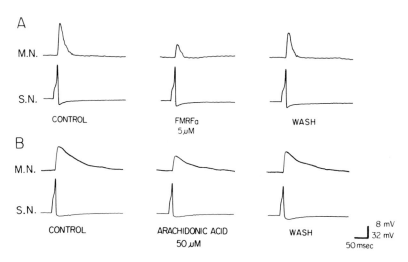

FIGURE 6.21. Arachidonic acid simulates FMRFamide-induced reduction in fast excitatory synaptic potential in follower motor neuron (M.N. traces) in response to firing an action potential in sensory neuron (S.N. traces). Records *A* (FMRFamide, 5 μmol/L) and *B* (arachidonic acid, 50 μmol/L) are from two different pairs of cells in intact abdominal ganglia. Reprinted by permission from *Nature* (1987); 328:38–43. Copyright © 1987 Macmillan Magazines Ltd.

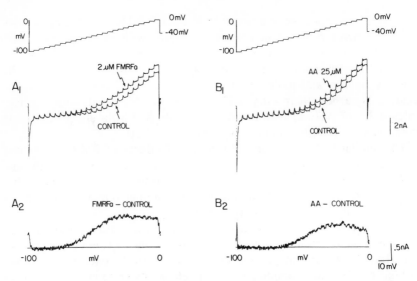

FIGURE 6.22. Comparison of the actions of FMRFamide and arachidonic acid on the total ionic current in voltage clamped sensory neurons. Effect of FMRFamide (2 μmol/L). Membrane potential held at -40 mV. Once every 30 seconds, a 50-ms staircase voltage command composed of 20-ms depolarizing steps of 4-mV increments, from -100 mV to 0 mV, was applied (upper left trace). A_1. Superimposed records of total membrane current before (lower trace, average of four records; control) and at peak action of the peptide (upper trace, average of two records, FMRFa). A_2. The control trace subtracted from the FMRFa trace to yield a FMRFamide-sensitive current. B_1 and B_2: current records from the same cell, after prolonged washing with normal seawater. B_1. Superimposed averaged records of total current before (average of five records) and during (average of two records) application of 25 μmol/L arachidonic acid. B_2. Arachidonic acid–sensitive current, obtained by subtraction of the records in B_1. Below -30 mV, it appears that the difference current largely reflects the outwardly rectifying S current. Positive to -30 mV contributions from other FMRFamide-sensitive currents (including a decreased calcium and calcium-activated K current) overlap with the S current (6,19,35–37). Reprinted by permission from *Nature* (1987); 328:38–43. Copyright © 1987 Macmillan Magazines Ltd.

FIGURE 6.23. Comparison of FMRFamide and arachidonic acid on single-S-channel currents. *A.* Single channel recordings from a cell-attached patch on a pleural sensory neuron in culture. Control record: before application of any compounds; +FMRFa: 7 minutes after application of 5 μmol/L FMRFamide to the bath; recovery: 20 minutes after washing the peptide out of the bath; +arachidonic acid: 6 minutes after application of 50 μmol/L arachidonic acid. Binomial fit to data yields estimate of $n=6$ for number of active S channels under all conditions. Records obtained at a patch potential depolarized by +80 mV above the resting potential. *B.* Effect of compounds on mean (time-averaged) current through patch. Mean current (I) measured from time integral of patch

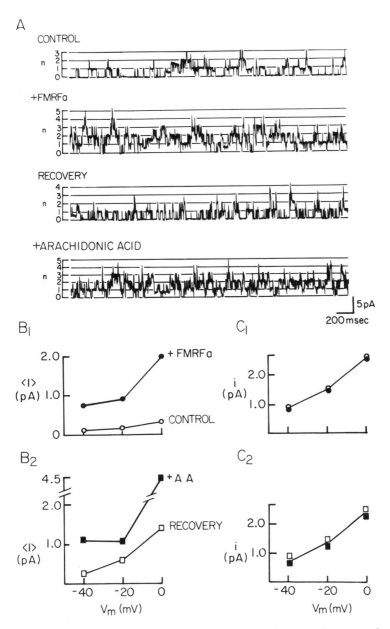

current above baseline for 30-second stretches of data at three membrane potentials. Membrane potential was altered from rest by changing voltage in the patch pipette. Voltages on abscissa are approximate transmembrane potentials of patch, assuming a resting potential of −60 mV. Current records were filtered at 500 Hz. *C*. Effects of compounds on single-channel current amplitude *i*. Symbols are same as those in *B*. Analysis in *B* and *C* is for experiment shown in *A*. Reprinted by permission from *Nature* (1987); 328:38–43. Copyright © 1987 Macmillan Magazines Ltd.

that of FMRFamide because it increases p, the channel-open probability, with no marked effect on N or i. Thus, by all the criteria we have tested, the actions of arachidonic acid and FMRFamide are identical.

Although these experiments show that arachidonic acid simulates the action of FMRFamide, they do not prove that metabolites of endogenous arachidonate mediate the response to the peptide. Arachidonic acid could be acting on the K^+ channel through an independent parallel mechanism. We have obtained evidence for an obligatory role of arachidonic acid using two separate approaches, one pharmacological and the other biochemical

Inhibitors of Arachidonic Acid Cascade Block
the Action of FMRFamide

The first step in the receptor-mediated generation of eicosanoids is the release of free arachidonate from membrane phospholipids, a reaction that in mammals is most commonly catalyzed by a phospholipase A_2, or by the combined action of phospholipase C and diacylglycerol lipase (31,38). Although selective inhibitors of either phospholipase are not yet available, both enzymes can be effectively blocked by 4-bromophenacyl bromide (32). This inhibitor, at a concentration of 10 μmol/L completely suppresses the hyperpolarization produced by FMRFamide in cultured neurons (Figure 6.24B) The fact that the depolarizing response to 5-HT is not affected in the same cells indicates that the drug does not interfere with S-channel function.

The experiments with the phospholipase inhibitor suggest that the release of arachidonic acid is a necessary step in the response to FMRFamide. To determine which metabolic pathway is responsible for producing the active eicosanoids, we tested the actions of indomethacin, which blocks cyclo-oxygenase (39) and nordihydroguaiaretic acid (NDGA), which blocks lipoxygenases (40) Indomethacin, which we find inhibits formation of prostaglandins in *Aplysia* ganglia with a half maximal inhibition concentration of 0.5 μmol/L without affecting lipoxygenase activity, has no effect on the hyperpolarization induced by FMRFamide (Figure 6.24C). By contrast, NDGA, which inhibits lipoxygenase activity in *Aplysia* nervous tissue with an IC_{50} of 3 μmol/L suppresses the hyperpolarizing response of sensory cells in culture to FMRFamide (Figure 6.24D). The depolarization produced by 5-HT was not affected. These experiments suggest that a lipoxygenase enzyme rather than cyclo-oxygenase is involved in the intracellular signaling process.

To determine whether lipoxygenase metabolites of arachidonic acid were actually released in response to FMRFamide, we studied clusters of sensory neurons dissected from pleural ganglia and labeled by incubation with (^{3}H)arachidonic acid. FMRFamide stimulates the formation of radioactive material that migrated on reversed-phase HPLC with authen-

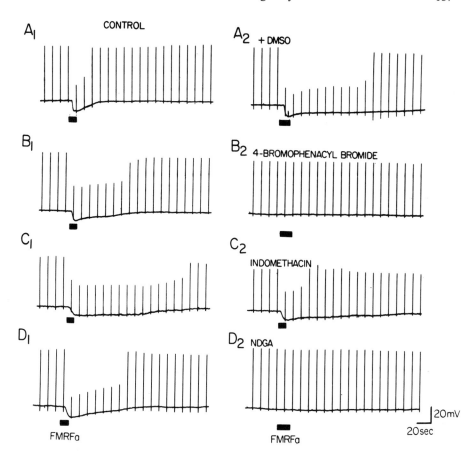

FIGURE 6.24. Actions of inhibitors of arachidonic acid metabolism on the response to FMRFamide. Chart records of membrane potential under current clamp from sensory cells in culture. Large, brief, upward deflections are action potentials elicited by depolarizing current pulses. Smaller upward deflections are the passive depolarizations following action potential blockade. The bars mark the application of 2 μmol/L FMRFamide onto the cell body. A–D are representative tracings from four experiments. The left-hand tracings (A_1–D_1) are control responses to the peptide recorded during continuous superfusion with artificial seawater (resting potential ranging between −38 and −57 mV). The right-hand tracings (A_2–D_2) are responses to a second application of FMRFamide on the same cells after superfusion of a test compound. A_2. After superfusion with dimethyl-sulfoxide in artificial seawater (DMSO, 1/10,000). B_2, C_2, D_2. After superfusion of the seawater-DMSO mixture, containing in addition: in B_2, the phospholipase inhibitor 4-bromophenacyl bromide (10 μmol/L); in C_2, the cyclo-oxygenase blocker indomethacin (5 μmol/L); in D_2, the lipoxygenase inhibitor nordihydro-guaiaretic acid (NDGA, 5 μmol/L) Reprinted by permission from *Nature* (1987); 328:38–43. Copyright © 1987 Macmillan Magazines Ltd.

tic 12-HETE and 5-HETE. A representative chromatogram is shown in
Figure 6.25 (upper panel). In control incubations (Figure 6.25, middle
panel) or incubations with artificial seawater containing 5-HT (Figure
6.25, lower panel) only background radioactivity was found in the
12-HETE and 5-HETE fractions.

12-HPETE Mimics the Action of FMRFamide

Independent support for the involvement of lipoxygenase metabolites
comes from experiments in which we directly tested the action of

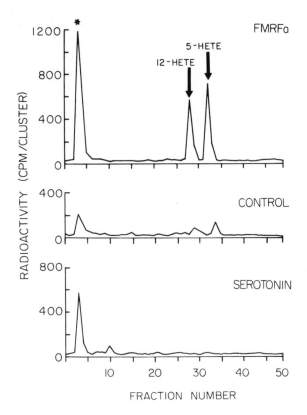

FIGURE 6.25. FMRFamide stimulates the release of lipoxygenase products from
sensory clusters of *Aplysia*. Representative reversed-phase HPLC fractionation
of samples from the incubation of one sensory cluster (200 cells) with 10 μmol/L
FMRFamide for 1 minute; (upper chromatogram), without FMRFamide (middle
chromatogram) or with 10 μmol/L 5-HT for 1 minute (lower chromatogram). The
arrows indicate the retention volumes of authentic 12-HETE and 5-HETE
standards. The radioactive material associated with the solvent front (*) was
consistently increased in the presence of FMRFamide. This component includes
polar metabolites of arachidonic acid that are not yet identified. Reprinted by
permission from *Nature* (1987); 328:38–43. Copyright © 1987 Macmillan Magazines Ltd.

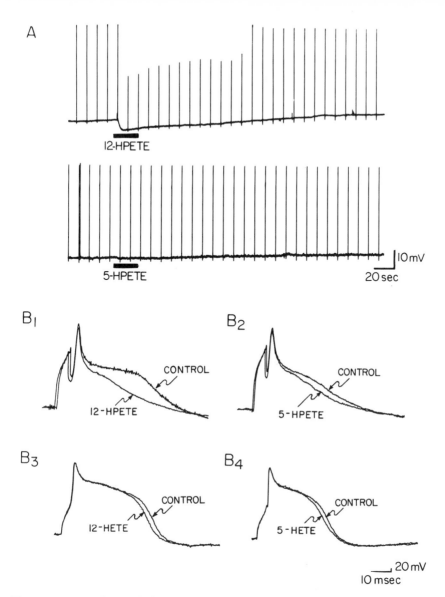

FIGURE 6.26. Effect of lipoxygenase metabolites on membrane and action potentials. *A.* Effect of 1.5 μmol/L 12-HPETE (top trace) and 1.5 μmol/L 5-HPETE (bottom trace) on resting potentials and stimulated action potentials (brief upward spikes) in pleural sensory neuron in culture. 12-HPETE inhibited spike firing for about 2 minutes: during this period the smaller spikes are subthreshold). Initial resting potential was −43 mV for top trace and −39 mV for bottom trace. B_2–B_4. Effects of metabolites on action potential duration recorded in 50 mmol/L TEA. Action potentials recorded from sensory neuron in intact abdominal ganglia. 12-HPETE and 5-HPETE (60 μmol/L) were applied to one cell while 12-HETE and 5-HETE (60 μmol/L) were applied to a second cell. Action potentials were elicited by brief depolarizing stimuli. In B_1 and B_2, the neuron fired a spike after termination of the brief current probe. Action potentials have been aligned to superimpose the rising phase. Reprinted by permission from *Nature* (1987); 328:38–43. Copyright © 1987 Macmillan Magazines Ltd.

exogenously applied arachidonic acid metabolites on the sensory neurons. Lipoxygenases convert arachidonate into hydroperoxy acids; in mammals these acids are either reduced to the corresponding hydroxy acids or transformed into metabolites that are distinctive for each of the lipoxygenase pathways (22). We tested the actions of both 12- and 5-hydroperoxy and hydroxy acids on the resting and action potentials of sensory neurons (Figure 6.26). Application of 12-HPETE (1.5 μmol/L) stimulates the slow hyperpolarization of the resting potential and the decrease in excitability seen with FMRFamide (Figure 6.26A). 5-HPETE, 5-HETE, and 12-HETE have little effect on resting potential (Figure 6.26A). Both 12-HPETE and 5-HPETE simulate the decrease in action potential duration observed with FMRFamide (Figure 6.26B). The average decrease in action potential duration with 12-HPETE, however, was two to three times greater than the decrease in response to 5-HPETE (Figure 6.26B_1, B_2). Again, 12-HETE and 5-HETE had little effect on the duration of the action potential (Figure 6.26 B_3, B_4). These results confirm the biochemical and pharmacological experiments that implicate lipoxygenase metabolites in the actions of FMRFamide; they further suggest that the active second messenger derives from a hydroperoxy acid rather than from a hydroxy acid.

An Overall View

Arachidonic Acid Cascade as A Second-Messenger System for Presynaptic Inhibition

We find that the receptor-stimulated release of arachidonic acid and its metabolism through a lipoxygenase pathway mediate the inhibitory synaptic response to the tetrapeptide FMRFamide in *Aplysia* sensory neurons. Our results provide direct evidence that lipoxygenase products act as second messengers in nerve cells and meet the criteria originally proposed for second-messenger systems by Robison, Butcher, and Sutherland (41).

1. *Synthesis.* The enzymatic machinery for producing lipoxygenase metabolites is present in neurons.
2. *Receptor mediation.* Formation of lipoxygenase metabolites is stimulated by applying the neuropeptide FMRFamide.
3. *Simulation.* Arachidonic acid and its lipoxygenase metabolites simulate the actions of FMRFamide.
4. *Selective blockade.* Agents that block arachidonic acid release and metabolism effectively inhibit the physiological response to FMRFamide.
5. *Termination.* Two mechanisms for terminating the action of the putative second messengers could be reduction to the inactive hydroxy acids and reincorporation into membrane phospholipids (30,41).

FMRFamide, Enkephalins, and the Modulation of Pain in the Mammalian Brain

A presynaptic inhibitory function for the arachidonic acid cascade probably is not unique to *Aplysia* sensory cells or to FMRFamide, since other experiments show that the presynaptic inhibition produced by stimulating the putative histaminergic L32 cells on the L10-RB connection (42) operates through the same second-messenger mechanism (30). It will be of interest to see whether arachidonic acid participates in presynaptic inhibition in vertebrates, such as that produced by enkephalins (43) and noradrenaline (44) in the dorsal root ganglion cells that mediate response to painful stimuli.

Arachidonic Acid Could Mediate Signals Between Neurons: The Case of LTP

Eicosanoids differ from other intracellular second messengers in one important way. Unlike other messengers, the eicosanoids are able to exit from the cell in which they are generated and act as first messengers on neighboring cells (45). As a result, a metabolite of arachidonic acid might provide a diffusible extracellular signal from a postsynaptic cell to a presynaptic one. This type of signal could explain the operation of a Hebbian type of synapse of the kind recently postulated to be important for long-term potentiation (LTP) of pyramidal cells in the CA_1 region of the hippocampus, where depolarization of the postsynaptic cell leads to enhanced release from the presynaptic region (46,47). In fact, Williams and Bliss (48) have recently tested this possibility and found that NDGA, the lipoxygenase inhibitor, blocks selectively the induction of LTP in the hippocampus CA_1 region, as well as in the dentate gyrus.

Inhibitory Override of Facilitation Occurs at the Level of the Kinase and Its Substrate Proteins

We have recently established that FMRFamide activation of the arachidonic acid cascade depends on a pertussis-toxin–sensitive G protein, which is likely to couple the peptide receptor to the phospholipase responsible for the release of arachidonate from sensory cell membrane phospholipids (21,49). From a functional point of view, this G protein seems not to be of the G_i kind, in that it does not significantly reverse adenylate cyclase activation. This finding adds further support to the earlier biochemical and biophysical evidence that, unlike the situation with transmitters utilizing G_i, where inhibitory override resides at the level of the G proteins and has adenylate cyclase activity as a target, the inhibition override produced by FMRFamide lies at a later stage in the cAMP cascade. This override involves either inhibition of the cAMP-dependent protein kinase or activation of a specific phosphatase that can reverse the phosphorylation process at the level of the same substrate proteins of cAMP-dependent kinase, or both. At the present time, we do not know whether the basic modulatory action of FMRFamide on the S channel (to increase the open probability) and its inhibition of 5-HT modulation (through reopening of the channels) share the same molecular mechanisms (eg, phosphatase activation) and are both mediated by the arachidonic acid pathway. Moreover, we have not yet identified the active lipoxygenase metabolite (or metabolites) ultimately responsible for S-channel modulation, although our results do suggest that the active molecule is closely related to a hydroperoxy acid, in particular to 12-HPETE. Whatever the answer to these questions, the inhibitory effect of FMRFamide acting through the eicosanoids is functionally antagonistic to the facilitatory action produced by 5-HT through cAMP. Since 5-HT and FMRFamide converge on the same K^+ channel, 5-HT to decrease and the peptide to increase channel activity, an individual channel protein can serve as a final common effector for different second-messenger systems.

Modulatory Systems and the Control of Synaptic Strength by Learning

Independent of the detailed biochemical modulation mechanisms, the experiments on learning indicated that the environment produces substantial effects on behavior by activating different modulatory systems. These modulatory systems act on nerve cells to regulate the cells' excitability and to control synaptic strength. Thus the action of the environment is represented in the brain by the activity in specific modulatory systems.

Presynaptic inhibition has two additional parallels to presynaptic facilitation. First, as is the case with presynaptic facilitation, presynaptic inhibition shows an activity-dependent enhancement. If the sensory neuron is active just before it is exposed to FMRFamide, the depression of transmitter release from the sensory neuron terminal is more powerful and more prolonged than if the sensory neuron is not active. This associative mechanism is characteristic of classical conditioning in the facilitating system and suggests that the inhibitory component may have a comparable role in the associative inhibitory conditioning. Second, repeated presentation of FMRFamide produces a long-term depression of transmitter release, which persists over 24 hours. Unlike the short-term process, which does not require new protein synthesis, this long-term process resembles the long-term facilitation produced by serotonin in being selectively blocked by inhibitors of protein synthesis. We have recently identified specific patterns of protein synthesis associated with long-term facilitation. It therefore also will be interesting to explore whether a comparable pattern of protein synthesis accompanies the turning on of the long-term inhibitory pathway.

In a larger sense, these studies of behavioral sensitization and inhibition illustrate that environmental contingencies can act on single sensory neurons through two different modulatory systems, one facilitatory and one inhibitory. These modulatory systems utilize two different families of transmitters (including serotonin for facilitation and FMRFamide for inhibition), and engage two different second-messenger systems within the sensory neurons—the cAMP cascade for facilitation and the lipoxygenase pathway of arachidonic acid for inhibition (Figure 6.27). Therefore, our results suggest that these opposing behavioral events are represented within the nervous system by the activation of antagonistic modulatory systems and are re-represented within single sensory neurons by the balance of actions of competing second-messenger systems. Thus, these results begin to reveal an unexpected richness at the cellular and molecular levels underlying the internal representation of external events.

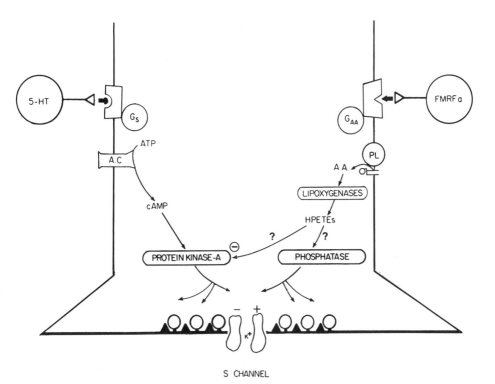

S CHANNEL

FIGURE 6.27. Proposed model for the molecular intracellular events leading to antagonistic modulation of the S K^+ channels in the sensory neurons of *Aplysia* by facilitatory (eg, 5-HT) and inhibitory (eg, FMRFamide) transmitters. The model is depicted in the synaptic terminal of the sensory neuron to emphasize the relevancy of these molecular events to the modulation by the environment of synaptic transmission in a circuit-mediating behavior.

References

1. Hille B (1984). *Ionic Channels of Excitable Membranes.* Sinauer, Sunderland, MA.
2. Castellucci VF, Schacher S, Montarolo PG, Mackey S, Glanzman DL, Hawkins RD, Abrams TW, Goelet P, Kandel ER (1986). Convergence of small molecule and peptide transmitters on a common molecular cascade. In T Hokfelt, K Fuxe, P Pernow, eds. *Coexistence of Neuronal Messengers: A New Principle in Chemical Transmission, Progress in Brain Research,* vol 68. Elsevier, New York, pp 83–102.
3. Schaefer M, Picciotto MR, Kreiner T, Kaldany TR, Taussig R, Scheller RD (1985). Aplysia neurons express a gene encoding multiple FMRFamide neuropeptides. *Cell* 41:457–467.
4. Comb M, Seeburg PH, Adelman J, Eiden L, Herbert H (1982). Primary structure of the human met- and leu-enkephalin precursor and its mRNA. *Nature (London)* 295:663–666.
5. Noda M, Furutani Y, Takahashi H, Toyosato M, Firose T, Inayam S, Nakanishi S, Numa S (1982). Cloning and sequence analysis of cDNA for bovine adrenal preproenkephalin. *Nature (London)* 295:202–206.
6. Belardetti F, Kandel ER, Siegelbaum S (1987). Neuronal inhibition by the peptide FMRFamide involves opening of S K^+ channels. *Nature (London)* 325:153–156.
7. Kandel ER, Schwartz JH (1982). Molecular biology of an elementary form of learning: Modulation of transmitter release by cyclic AMP. *Science* 218: 433–443.
8. Castellucci VF, Kandel ER, Schwartz JH, Wilson FD, Nairn AC, Greengard P (1980). Intracellular injection of the catalytic subunit of cyclic AMP-dependent protein kinase simulates facilitation of transmitter release underlying behavioral sensitization in *Aplysia. Proc Natl Acad Sci USA* 77:7492–7496.
9. Shuster MJ, Camardo JS, Siegelbaum SA, Kandel ER (1985). Cyclic AMP-dependent protein kinase closes the serotonin-sensitive K^+ channels of *Aplysia* sensory neurones in cell-free membrane patches. *Nature (London)* 313:392–395.
10. Klein M, Kandel ER (1978). Presynaptic modulation of voltage-dependent Ca^{2+} current: Mechanism for behavioral sensitization in *Aplysia californica. Proc Natl Acad Sci Usa* 75:3512–3516.
11. Klein M, Camardo JS, Kandel ER (1982). Serotonin modulates a specific potassium current in the sensory neurons that show presynaptic facilitation in *Aplysia. Proc Natl Acad Sci USA* 79:5713–5717.
12. Klein M, Hochner B, Kandel ER (1986). Facilitatory transmitters and cAMP can modulate accommodation as well as transmitter release in *Aplysia* sensory neurons: Evidence for parallel processing in a single cell. *Proc Natl Acad Sci USA* 83:7994–7998.
13. Hochner B, Klein M, Schacher S, Kandel ER (1986). Action potential duration and the modulation of transmitter release from the sensory neurons of *Aplysia* in presynaptic facilitation and behavioral sensitization. *Proc Natl Acad Sci USA* 83:8410–8414.

14. Hochner B, Klein M, Schacher S, Kandel ER (1986). Additional component in the cellular mechanism of presynaptic facilitation contributes to behavioral dishabituation in *Aplysia*. *Proc Natl Acad Sci USA* 83:8794–8798.
15. Boyle MB, Klein K, Smith SJ, Kandel ER (1984). Serotonin increases intracellular Ca^{2+} transients in voltage-clamped sensory neurons of *Aplysia californica*. *Proc Natl Acad Sci USA* 81:7642–7646.
16. Hochner B, Schacher S, Klein M, Kandel ER (1985). Presynaptic facilitation in *Aplysia* sensory neurons: A process independent of K^+ current modulation becomes important when transmitter release is depressed. *Soc Neurosci Abstr* 11:29.
17. Siegelbaum SA, Camardo JS, Kandel ER (1982). Serotonin and cyclic AMP close single K^+ channels in *Aplysia* sensory neurones. *Nature (London)* 299:413–417.
18. Siegelbaum SA, Tsien RW (1983). Modulation of gated ion channels as a mode of transmitter action. *Trends Neurosci* 6:307–313.
19. Brezina V, Eckert R, Erxleben C (1987). Modulation of potassium conductances by an endogenous neuropeptide in neurones of *Aplysia californica*. *J Physiol* 382:267–290.
20. Brezina V, Eckert R, Erxleben C (1987). Suppression of calcium current by an endogenous neuropeptide in neurones of *Aplysia californica*. *J Physiol* 388:565–596.
21. Volterra A, Siegelbaum SA (1988). Role of two different quanine nucleotide-binding proteins in the antagonistic modulation of the S-type K^+ channel by cAMP and arachidonic acid metabolites in Aplysia sensory neurons. *Proc Natl Acad Sci USA* 85:7810–7814.
22. Ocorr KA, Byrne JH (1985). Membrane responses and changes in cAMP levels in *Aplysia* sensory neurons produced by serotonin, tryptamine, FMRFamide, and small cardioactive peptide B (SCP_B). *Neurosci Lett* 55:113–118.
23. Needleman P, Turk J, Jakschick BA, Morrison AR, Lefkowith JB (1986). Arachidonic acid metabolisms. *Ann Rev Biochem* 55:69–102.
24. Samuelsson B (1964). Identification of a smooth muscle-stimulating factor in bovine brain. *Biochem Biophys Acta* 84:218–219.
25. Sautebin L, Spagnuolo C, Galli C, Galli G (1978). A mass fragmentographic procedure for the simultaneous determination of HETE and PGF_{2alpha} in the central nervous system. *Prostaglandins* 16:985–988.
26. Wolfe LS (1982). Eicosanoids: Prostaglandins, thromboxanes, leukotrienes and other derivatives of carbon-20 unsaturated fatty acids. *J Neurochem* 38:1–14.
27. Lindgren JA, Hokfelt T, Dahlen SE, Patrono C, Samuelsson B (1984). Leukotrienes in the rat central nervous system. *Proc Natl Acad Sci USA* 81:6212–6216.
28. Shimizu T, Takusagawa Y, Izumi T, Ohishi N & Seyama Y (1987). Enzymic synthesis of leukotriene B_4 in guinea pig brain. *J Neurochem* 48:1541–1546.
29. Piomelli D, Volterra A, Dale N, Siegelbaum SA, Kandel ER, Schwartz JH, Belardetti F (1987). Lipoxygenase metabolites of arachidonic acid as second messengers for presynaptic inhibition of *Aplysia* sensory cells. *Nature (London)* 328:38–43.

30. Piomelli D, Shapiro E, Feinmark SJ, Schwartz JH (1987). Metabolites of arachidonic acid in the nervous system of *Aplysia:* Possible mediators of synaptic modulation. *J Neurosci* 7:3675–3686.
31. Van den Bosch (1980). Intracellular phospholipase A. *Biochem Biophys Acta* 604:191–246.
32. Blackwell GJ, Flower RJ (1983). Inhibition of phospholipase. *Brit Med Bull* 39:260–264.
33. Pace-Asciak CR, Granstrom E, Samuelsson B (1983). Arachidonic acid epoxides. Isolation and structure of two hydroxy epoxide intermediates in the formation of 8,11,12- and 10,11,12-trihydroxy eicosatrienoic acids. *J Biol Chem* 258:6835–6840.
34. Choi DW, Fischbach GD (1981). GABA conductance of chick spinal cord and dorsal root ganglion neurons in cell culture. *J Neurophysiol* 45:605–620.
35. Colombaioni L, Paupardin-Tritsch D, Vidal PP, Gerschenfeld HM (1985). The neuropeptide FMRFamide decreases both the Ca^{2+} conductance and a cyclic $3',5'$-adenosine monophosphate-dependent K^+ conductance in identified Helix neurons. *J Neurosci* 5:2533–2538.
36. Ruben P, Johnson JW, Thompson S (1986). Analysis of FMRF-amide effect on *Aplysia* bursting neurons. *J Neurosci* 6:252–259.
37. Cottrell GA, Davies NW, Green KA (1984). Multiple actions of a molluscan cardioexcitatory neuropeptide and related peptides on identified Helix neurones. *J Physiol* 356:315–333.
38. Irvine RF (1982). How is the level of free arachidonic acid controlled in mammalian cells? *Biochem J* 204:3–16.
39. Shen TY, Winter CA (1977). Chemical and biological studies on indomethacin, sulindac and their analogs. *Advances Drug Res* 12:89–245.
40. Salari H, Braquet P, Borgeat P (1984). Comparative effects of indomethacin, acetylenic acids, 15-HETE, nodihydroguaiaretic acid and BW 755 C on the metabolism of arachidonic acid in human leukocytes and platelets. *Prostaglandins Leukotrienes Med* 13:53–60.
41. Robison GA, Butcher RW, Sutherland EQ (1971). *Cyclic AMP* Academic Press, Orlando, FL.
42. Kretz R, Shapiro E, Kandel ER (1986). Presynaptic inhibition produced by an identified presynaptic inhibitory neuron. I. Physiological mechanisms. *J Neurophysiol* 55:131–146.
43. Mudge A, Leeman S, Fischbach GD (1979). Enkephalin inhibits release of substance P from sensory neurons in culture and decreases action potential duration. *Proc Natl Acad Sci USA* 76:526–530.
44. Dunlap K, Fischbach GD (1978). Neurotransmitters decrease the calcium component of sensory neuron action potentials. *Nature (London)* 276:837–838.
45. Hedqvist P (1977). Basic mechanisms of prostaglandin action on autonomic neurotransmission. *Ann Rev Pharmacol Toxicol* 17:259–279.
46. Wigstrom H, Gustafson B, Huang Y-Y, Abraham WD (1986). Hippocampal long-lasting potentiation is induced by pairing single afferent volley with intracellular injected depolarizing current pulses. *Acta Physiol Scand* 126:317–319.
47. Bliss TVP, Douglas RM, Errington MC, Lynch MA (1986). Correlation

between long-term potentiation and release of endogenous amino acids from denate gyrus of anesthetized cats. *J Physiol* 377:391–408.

48. Williams, Bliss TVP (1988). Induction but not maintenance of calcium-induced long-term potentiation in dentate gyrus and area CA₁ of the hippocampal slice is blocked by nordihydroguaiaretic acid. *Neurosci Lett* 88:81–85.

49. Volterra A, Sweatt JD, Siegelbaum SA (1987). Involvement of G proteins in the inhibitory action of FMRFamide through lipoxygenase metabolities of arachidonic acid in *Aplysia* sensory neurons. *Soc Neurosci Abstr* 13:1440.

CHAPTER 7

Applications of Molecular Genetics to Neuropsychiatric Disorders

Joseph B. Martin

The pace of discovery following the applications of molecular genetics to the clinical neurosciences has been astonishing. A decade ago, knowledge of the causes of the many genetic disorders that affect the central nervous system (CNS) was limited to a few autosomal recessive lysosomal storage diseases. The approaches to understanding these disorders used classic protein chemistry to isolate enzymes shown to be active in catabolism of brain lipids. The absence of specific enzymes was shown to be the cause of the lipid storage diseases in question.

Advances in the Autosomal Recessive Diseases

In recent years several of the defective enzymes that cause these autosomal recessive diseases have been cloned and their chromosomal localizations identified. The best characterized of this group are Tay-Sachs disease and Sandhoff disease (GM_2 gangliosidoses). Both diseases are lipid storage disorders caused by mutations in the α or β chains, respectively, of the enzyme β-hexosaminidase [1–3]. Two isoenzymes of hexosaminidase are known: type A, which is composed of one α- and two β-chains, and type B, composed of four β-chains. The α-chain is encoded on chromosome 15 and the β-chain on chromosome 5. Tay-Sachs disease, which is caused by a mutation in the α-chain, is characterized during the first year of life by mental retardation, cherry-red spot in the macula of the eye, and seizures. There is no hepatosplenomegaly. Sandhoff disease, resulting from a defect in the β-chain, has a similar clinical picture, with the added feature of lipid-laden foam cells in the bone marrow. The molecular basis of the two diseases has now been partially elucidated. Both the gene for the α-chain [2] and that for the β-chain [3] have been cloned. They are ancestrally related with about 50% homology. The genes contain 14 exons spanning nearly 50 kilobases.

Tay-Sachs disease is associated in families of Ashkenazi Jewish origin with defective α-chain messenger RNA in fibroblasts [2]. Allelic heterogeneity of the genetic defect has been found by comparison of these lineages with others of French-Canadian ancestry. In the latter, a different mutation has been defined, in which a 5' deletion of approximately 5 to 8 kb occurs in the gene encoding for the α-chain, whereas in Ashkenazi Jewish patients there is an intact gene. Sandhoff disease also shows genetic heterogeneity, with a distinction reported for cases of infantile versus juvenile onset. In 4 of 11 infantile cases, deficiencies in pre-β-chain mRNA were detected and found to be associated with partial gene deletions in the 5' end of the gene on chromosome 5. In juvenile cases, normal or reduced levels of pre-β-chain mRNA were found with no abnormalities in the Hex B gene. These data indicate that each clinical subgroup of either Tay-Sachs or Sandhoff disease is associated with different Hex A or B mutations, respectively.

Another systemic lipid storage disease, Gaucher's disease, is caused by a deficiency in the lysosomal enzyme glucocerebrosidase (1). The disease is classified clinically into three subtypes: 1, 2, and 3. The CNS is not involved in type 1. Type 2, a rarer form, appears in the first 6 months of life as a rapidly progressive neuronopathic storage disease; clinical features include cranial nerve and brainstem abnormalities and marked hepatosplenomegaly. In type 3, nervous system degeneration occurs later in life and progression in slower. The molecular basis of the enzymatic defect in type 2 has recently been postulated. Tsuji et al (4) discovered a single-base pair change (T to C) on chromosome 1, which led to substitution of proline for leucine in amino acid position 444 of glucocerebrosidase. This change resulted in a new cleavage site for the restriction endonuclease NciI. It was speculated that this single–amino acid mutation affects the α-helical structure of the enzyme, resulting in inactivation. The new cleavage site provided the opportunity to use restriction fragment length variations generated by NciI digests to detect homozygotes and unaffected heterozygotes in pedigrees of affected families. An unexpected finding was that not all type 2 patients were homozygous for the defect. Not surprising, none of the type 1 patients was homozygous. These findings are of considerable interest in pointing out how minor mutations can cause devastating diseases but leave unanswered how molecular differences can account for the variable phenotypic expression between types 1, 2, and 3.

These disorders illustrate progress made using the conventional approach of molecular genetics—that is, to identify the abnormal protein, define its mRNA, and locate the gene encoding for it.

DNA RFLP Markers for Diseases of the Nervous System

Discovering an approach to defining the genetic basis for autosomal dominant and X-linked recessive disorders has taken a different path. It was first proposed by Botstein, White, and colleagues in 1980 (5) that

TABLE 7.1. Chromosomal localization and gene abnormalities in selected neurological diseases

Genetic classification and Disease	Chromosome	Gene defect	Comments on genetic heterogeneity
Autosomal dominant			
Huntington's disease	4p16.3	Unknown	None demonstrated in over 100 pedigrees
Myotonic dystrophy	19 centromere	Unknown	None demonstrated
Familial Alzheimer's disease	21q21	Unknown (not by amyloid)	Not adequately studied
Familial amyloidotic polyneuropathy	18q11.2-q12.1	Single–base pair substitution in mRNA for transthyretin	Allelic heterogeneity
Manic-depressive illness	11p.Xp	Unknown	Evidence for nonallelic heterogeneity
Spinocerebellar atrophy	6	Unknown	Unknown
Von Recklinghausen's neurofibromatosis (NFI)	17q-centrome	Unknown	None demonstrated in over 25 pedigrees
Bilateral acoustic neurofibromatosis (NFII)	22q	Unknown	Unknown
Charcot-Marie-Tooth disease (type 1)	1q2	Unknown	Unknown
X-linked recessive			
Duchenne dystrophy	Xp21.21	Absence of dystrophin	Multiallelic heterogeneity
Becker dystrophy	Xp21.21	Defect in dystrophin	Unknown

Disease	Location	Molecular defect	Heterogeneity
Adrenoleukodystrophy	Xq27-q28	Unknown	Multiallelic heterogeneity
Lesch-Nyhan syndrome	Xq27	HPRT deficiency, variations	
Pelizaeus-Merzbacher disease	Xq21-q22	Defect in myelin proteolipid protein	Unknown
Autosomal recessive			
Gaucher's disease	1q21	Amino acid substitution in glucocerebrosidase	Allelic heterogeneity
G_{M2} gangliosidosis			
Tay-Sachs disease (type 1)	15q22-q25	Mutation in gene encoding chain of hexosaminidase	Allelic heterogeneity
Sandhoff disease (type 2)	5q13	Mutation in gene encoding chain of hexosaminidase	Allelic heterogeneity
Wilson's disease	13q14.11	Unknown (not ceruloplasmin)	Unknown
Recessive with germinal chromosomal deletion			
Central neurofibromatosis	22q11-q13	Unknown	Unknown
Retinoblastoma	13q14	Partially characterized	Allelic heterogeneity
Meningioma	22q12.3-qter	Unknown	Unknown
Von Hippel-Lindau disease	3p	Unknown	Unknown

Revised and reprinted from J. B. Martin (1987). *Science* 238:765–771, with permission. Copyright 1987 by the AAAS.

restriction fragment length polymorphisms (RFLPs) are sufficiently abundant in human DNA to make them useful for DNA linkage studies to determine the location of genes for any autosomal dominant disorder. This notion, also advocated by Housman and Gusella in 1981 (6) has proved to be an accurate prediction; to date more than a dozen human diseases affecting the nervous system have been assigned to individual chromosomes using this technique (Table 7.1). In the case of the X-linked disorders, particularly those associated with cytogenetic abnormalities, such as Duchenne's dystrophy, it has been possible to locate the entire gene and its protein product by a process commonly referred to as "reverse genetics." This review updates recent advances in this area.

Genetic Linkage Analysis with RFLPs

In order to define the chromosomal map position of a gene causing an autosomal dominant disorder it is first necessary to assemble large pedigrees affected by the disorder in whom it is possible to segregate definitively those affected by the disease (gene carriers) from those unaffected (7,8). Because only a small portion of the total human genome has been mapped using known genes for proteins (A, B, and O blood groups, hemoglobin genes, human lymphocyte antigens, oncogenes, etc), a strategy of using anonymous or identified DNA probes to cover

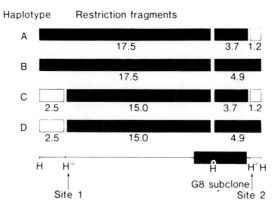

FIGURE 7.1. Haplotypes at the G8 locus. The G8 marker results from the detection of two polymorphic Hind III sites, each giving two possible alleles (presence of the site or absence of the site). The combination of alleles from each of these tightly linked sites is referred to as a haplotype. At the G8 locus, there are four possible haplotypes: A, B, C, and D. The subclone of G8 used as probe (pK082) is depicted and the fragments it detects for each haplotype are shaded. The unshaded fragments are also characteristic of each haplotype but are not overlapping with the probe and therefore are not seen on hybridization. Reprinted from reference 7, with permission.

intervals of the entire genome was necessary. In the space of a few years, more than 2,000 DNA probes have been identified and many have been assigned to specific chromosomes. The values of such probes in genetic linkage analysis is the ability to use them as inherited markers close to the disease gene. Such linkage offers an immediate opportunity for presymptomatic or prenatal genetic testing and is the first step toward isolation of the abnormal gene itself.

The basic tool of recombinant DNA technology is the restriction endonuclease, which cuts double-stranded DNA at specific base sequences. A small alteration, even a single base pair substitution (or mutation) located in the DNA at one of these recognition sequences, prevents enzymatic cleavage at that site (Figures 7.1 and 7.2). RFLPs

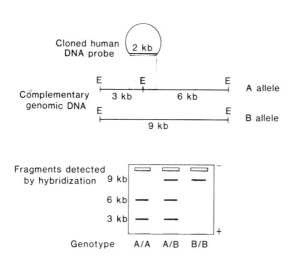

FIGURE 7.2. Restriction fragment length polymorphism (RFLP). In this example of an RFLP, a cloned 2-kb single-copy sequence of human DNA is capable of detecting the presence or absence of a polymorphic Eco RI (E) site. The presence of the variable site results in Eco RI fragments of 3 and 6 kb, the A allele at this locus. The B allele results when the central Eco RI site is missing because of the absence of the exact recognition sequence GAATTC. This site could have been lost as a result of a single base change in the genomic DNA. The B allele is recognized by a 9-kb ECO RI fragment. Individuals can be typed at the marker locus by digesting their genomic DNA to completion with Eco RI, resolving the DNA fragments by agarose gel electrophoresis, transferring the DNA from the gel to a solid filter support and hybridizing with the radioactive probe. The position at which the probe hybridizes to a complementary sequence is then detected by autoradiography. The inset shows the pattern observed for each of three possible genotypes at the marker locus. If the probe molecule did not cross the variable Eco RI site but was derived totally from the region of the 6-kb fragment, then the A and B alleles would be the 6-kb fragment and 9-kb fragment, respectively. The 3-kb fragment would therefore not be detected by the probe in this situation. Reprinted from reference 7, with permission.

generated by this difference are inherited and, if close enough to a defective gene, can be employed as markers for linkage to the disease in question.

Huntington's Disease

Huntington's disease (HD), an autosomal dominant disorder, was the first of the human genetic disorders in which the gene location was discovered by RFLPs and linkage analysis (9,10). HD manifests itself clinically with a progressive involuntary movement disorder, psychiatric changes, particularly depression, and (in the later stages) profound dementia. The age of onset in most cases is between 25 and 45 years, but early-onset juvenile cases, more frequently inherited from the father, also occur. Late-onset cases are also described, with clinical symptoms beginning in the sixth to eighth decades. In these latter cases, the disease is mild, the dementia is moderate, and inheritance more often is transmitted via the mother.

Recent investigations of the neuropathology of HD have shown the principal abnormalities to be in the neurons that project from the striatum to other regions of the basal ganglia (11). A severe atrophy occurs in the caudate and putamen as a result of the loss of nerve cells. There is also atrophy in the cerebral cortex, although the precise neuronal changes that result in tissue loss there remain ill defined. In the striatum it has been demonstrated that *spiny* cells containing the neurotransmitters γ-aminobutyric acid (GABA), substance P, the enkephalins, and dynorphin are affected severely, whereas local interneurons of the *aspiny* type, which contain somatostatin, and neuropeptide Y are spared. This differential effect, which can be mimicked in animals by administration of neurotoxic agents that interact with *N*-methyl-*D*-aspartate receptors, has provided one hypothesis concerning a role of endogenous excitotoxins, such as quinolinic acid, in causing the cell loss (12,13).

Genetic linkage studies using a probe located on the short arm of chromosome 4 [G8 probe, locus D4S10] (14) have now been studied in more than 100 pedigrees worldwide. These studies show positive linkage without any reported exception and support the impression from clinical and epidemiological studies that Huntington's disease may have originated from a single mutation that occurred 400 or 500 years ago. Subsequent studies have revealed additional polymorphisms at this locus. It is currently estimated that the D4S10 locus resides about 4 to 5 million base pairs proximal to the HD gene locus (15). D4S10 has been physically mapped to 4p16.3, the terminal region of chromosome 4, estimated to comprise about 3% of the chromosome (16). The newest probe, C4H(D4S43) is closer to the HD gene than D4S10. It was defined by analysis of a 3.0-kb single-copy Hind III fragment derived from a chromosome 4–specific library (17). RFLPs isolated from this region of chromosome 4 in a cosmid clone and analyzed by multipoint analysis show that C4H(D4S43) lies between G8 and the HD gene and both are proximal to the HD locus. The HD gene is now estimated to lie 1–1.5 million base pairs from the telomere; despite saturation of the 4p region with more than 100 chromosome 4–specific probes, none has so far been genetically or physically mapped to the other side of the HD locus; that is, no flanking marker has yet been found. Initial speculations that genes found within and adjacent to the D4S43 locus might be candidate genes for HD (17) have now been quashed by identification of several recombinations between the HD locus and the D4S43 locus. These recombinations suggest that this locus is approximately 1–1.5 million base pairs away from the HD gene.

The possibility exists that the HD gene may represent a fixed translocation from another chromosomal site that has been inherited intact from generation to generation. Efforts are under way currently to clone DNA in cosmid or yeast vectors from the entire 4p16.3 region. The identification of the HD gene is likely to involve considerable additional effort. It is estimated that between 10 and 20 genes might reside in this region, and it will be no small experimental accomplishment to locate and recognize the abnormal gene.

HD in the Homozygous Gene State

Some additional observations concerning mechanisms of autosomal dominant inheritance have arisen with studies in Huntington's disease. It is now known that individuals in the Venezuelan pedigree, recognized by DNA linkage studies to be homozygous for HD, show identical clinical manifestations as do individuals who are heterozygous (18). It appears that HD is an example of genetically documented true dominance in which complete phenotypic dominance occurs with a single mutant allele. Such complete dominance by a single gene has been studied in *Drosophila* and in *C. elegans* and is hypothesized to be associated with mutations that cause a gain of function, meaning that the mutation may be deleterious by *expressing a normal cellular function in excess*. This concept is important because it raises the possibility that therapeutic strategies might be directed at suppressing the gene function in HD to prevent or retard the progress of the disease as opposed to the much more difficult issue of replacing a deficient gene function.

Presymptomatic Testing of HD

The discovery of DNA markers linked to the HD gene has given rise to the possibility of presymptomatic or predictive testing for the disease (Figure 7.3). Such studies have now been undertaken at several centers, and we have recently reported on our experience in several families in the

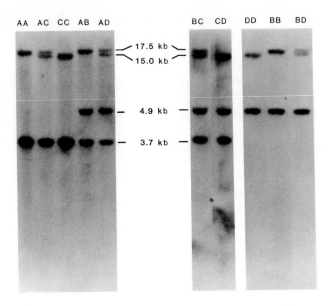

FIGURE 7.3. Autoradiograph showing each of the ten possible genotypes at the G8 locus. The pattern of fragments observed for each combination of haplotypes can be predicted from this illustration. The pattern observed for the gentoype AD is identical to that for BC; they can be distinguished only by typing close relatives of the individual with the ambiguous genotype. Reprinted from reference 7, with permission.

New England area (19). The first test results involved identifying the allele or forms of the DNA marker (D4S10) that is genetically linked to the Huntington's disease gene in each family and to use information obtained from affected and unaffected living members (or from frozen brain preserved at autopsy) to make predictions about the carrier state of the individual at risk. Because it is a linkage test and not a specific-gene test, it requires the cooperation of family members and the ascertainment of the particular DNA marker in each respective family. Moreover, since there is a calculated 4% chance of recombination between the D4S10 locus and the HD gene, the test is not absolutely accurate. An informative test can be used to adjust the probability of inheriting the Huntington's disease gene from 50% to a much higher or lower figure, but never greater than 96% to 98%.

In our studies, 47 participants entered the study from a total population inquiring about the test that numbered over 200. Of the 47 participants, 18 withdrew voluntarily after an initial visit to receive information about the test. Another individual met primary criteria for exclusion based on psychiatric grounds and withdrew after being informed of the reasons for not proceeding with the test. One family was too small to permit an analysis, five individuals were diagnosed for the first time as symptomatic of Huntington's disease, and 16 test results were given, 15 to adults and one prenatal test. Of these 16, four were positive, seven were negative, and five were uninformative. We anticipate that the use of the C4H probe will improve these analyses by increasing the likelihood of heterozygosity in those individuals who were uninformative because of a homozygous polymorphism. Our experience in following these patients after the test results indicates that individuals who tested positive not unexpectedly experienced intermittent depression, but none required hospitalization and no suicidal threats were reported. Our experience indicates that a presymptomatic test, though imperfect, can be given with appropriate clinical precautions and that no outstanding adverse effects have occurred thus far.

Alzheimer's Disease

Alzheimer's disease (AD), first described in 1906 by Alois Alzheimer, is a neurodengenerative disorder characterized by memory loss and other disorders of cognitive function (20). Neuropathological changes include intraneuronal neurofibrillary tangles and senile (neuritic) plaques. The latter contain a central core of extracellular amyloid surrounded by degenerating distended neuronal processes.

Substantial advances in understanding the nature of this condition have occurred during the past 2 years. These studies have resulted in the location of the gene in familial Alzheimer's disease (FAD), which is inherited as an autosomal dominant trait, to chromosome 21 and to the cloning of the gene for the amyloid protein. About 10% of patients with typical Alzheimer's disease, often with an earlier or presenile onset, inherit the disorder in a well-defined autosomal dominant pattern. This has been an important subgroup to study. The application of RFLPs located on chromosome 21 probes led to the demonstration in four families that the gene for FAD resides with close linkage to two probes (designated D21S1/D21S11) within the proximal region of the long arm of chromosome 21 (21). A group of DNA probes to this region was chosen after recognition that brains from patients with Down's syndrome (trisomy 21) who live past the fourth decade invariably manifest the same neuropathological features as seen in AD, including both neurofibrillary tangles and senile plaques.

The identification of the gene for the amyloid protein was accomplished by classic genetics using the amino acid sequence derived from cerebral vascular (β-amyloid) and neuritic plaque amyloid (A4 amyloid), both of which have a similar structure (22,23). Oligonucleotide probes constructed from the known amino acid sequence were used independently in four laboratories to clone the gene (24–27). The fact that the gene for amyloid was shown to be located on chromosome 21 caused the initial speculation that the etiology of Alzheimer's disease had been discovered.

However, the identification of the complementary DNA (cDNA) encoding for the amyloid protein has resulted in the recognition that the protein is a normal protein expressed not only in the brain but also in kidney, thymus, muscle, heart, and liver (27). Kang and co-workers (26) described a full-length cDNA encoding for a large precursor protein of the amyloid peptide. They speculated, based upon its structure, that it might be an intrinsic membrane protein. Initial studies suggested that gene duplication with excessive β-amyloid production might occur in sporadic Alzheimer's disease, as has been shown to occur in Down's syndrome with trisomy 21 (28). However, subsequent experiments from several laboratories have failed to confirm this finding and it now seems proven that the amyloid protein is not produced in excess in either FAD or sporadic AD in any tissues of the body, including brain (29–31). *In situ* hybridization studies have shown the amyloid message to be located in neurons in several brain regions and also in brain vessels (32).

A recent discovery reported simultaneously from two laboratories indicates that alternate RNA splicing may produce another amyloid-associated protein of larger size, which has resident within it a structure consistent with the Kunitz family of serine protease inhibitors (33,34). This new discovery, which was followed by demonstration of a different distribution of the alternate mRNA in brain and in peripheral tissues (34), has led to theories concerning a pathogenetic mechanism for amyloid deposition—that abnormalities of protein degradation may be involved in Alzheimer's disease. These ideas remain entirely speculative at the present time.

Genetic linkage studies of probes on chromosome 21 have shown clearly that the β-amyloid gene locus is distal to the FAD gene and indicate that the two loci are separated by at least 10–15 centimorgans (cM). At this juncture the significance of the amyloid deposition (ie, whether it is a cause or a result of the disease) remains unknown. It remains controversial, for example, whether the amyloid in brain is of peripheral or brain origin. Because it is present in cerebral blood vessels as well as in senile plaques (and, as shown by one group, may also be present in neurofibrillary tangles purified from neurons), any hypothesis remains plausible.

Although linkage has been demonstrated in four families of FAD, the possibility of genetic nonallelic heterogeneity cannot be excluded until many more families are studied. So far the markers identified by St. George-Hyslop et al (21) have not been used for presymptomatic recognition of the disease in these families.

Duchenne Dystrophy

The application of "reverse genetics"—that is, going from a defective gene to discover the abnormal cellular protein for which it encodes—has now been accomplished in Duchenne muscular dystrophy (DMD), the most common of the childhood dystrophies, which is inherited as an X-linked recessive disorder. The incidence is approximately 1 in 3,500 newborn boys; at least one-third of cases represent new mutations (35). The disease is recognized in the early years of life by muscle weakness and muscle fiber necrosis, accompanied by elevation in blood levels of the muscle enzyme creatine phosphokinase. Mental retardation occurs in 30% of DMD-afflicted males.

The DMD gene has been localized to the middle of the short arm of the X chromosome in band Xp21 by mapping chromosomal deletions associated with the disease in males, by isolating the junction fragment from a translocation (X;21) in a female with DMD, and by linkage to cloned anonymous probes containing RFLPs in adjacent DNA sequences (36–40). The development of multiple extragenic and intragenic probes with RFLPs has improved markedly the accuracy of gene diagnosis in female carriers and in prenatal at-risk males, although the high mutation rate has complicated such analyses (41). Pitfalls in accurate diagnosis of the gene defect result also from the large size of the DMD gene and from crossover events. It is now known, on the basis of RFLP linkage analysis and the identification of the abnormal protein in Duchenne dystrophy that the less severe and less common Becker variant (incidence 1 in 30,000, onset in late childhood or early adulthood) is caused by an abnormality at the same gene locus.

Physical restriction maps, generated by pulsed-field gradient gel electrophoresis, cover the Xp21 gene locus over a region containing up to a total of 3 million bp. The positions of several probes linked to DMD have been assigned to this physical map, which covers approximately 2% of the X chromosome (42).

To define precisely the region containing the defective gene in DMD, Monaco and co-workers (39,40) used subtraction hybridization techniques to clone sequences within a large deletion spanning the DMD locus. One cloned DNA segment, pERT87, detected deletions in 5% to 10% of DMD patients. Subclones of pERT87 were used to initiate chromosome walking in genomic phage libraries. A segment of genomic DNA (220 kb, designated the DXS164 locus) was isolated, and it contained sequences that were deleted or altered in males with DMD. In a large international collaborative study, 6.5% of males (88 of 1,346) with DMD or the Becker variant were found to have complete or partial deletions of the DXS164 locus. One observation made in these studies of the DXS164 locus was the frequent recombination rate (4% to 6%) within the DMD gene, suggesting that the DMD locus was unusually large. Complete cloning of the gene has now confirmed that it encompasses at least 60 exons spanning more than 2000 kb.

To find exons in the DXS164 locus, Monaco et al (40) used single-copy genomic clones to hybridize to Southern blots from a variety of mammalian species. One clone, which hybridized to the DNA of several mammals tested, hybridized to a large transcript of RNA isolated from human fetal skeletal muscle. From this RNA, cDNA clones were isolated that covered approximately 10% of the transcript.

The large protein that is encoded by the DMD gene has a molecular weight of over 400 kilodaltons (41). The protein, novel in structure, has been designated *dystrophin*. Antibodies to it show a subcellular location at the T-system/sarcoplasmic reticulum triad, where dystrophin is presumed to be a membrane-attached structural protein (42–44). The protein is absent in human dystrophic muscle from patients with Duchenne dystrophy and is altered in molecular size in patients with Becker dystrophy, probably because of a frame shift in DNA encoding for the protein. The protein has been shown to be expressed in normal muscle maintained in culture and to be absent in muscles cultured from Duchenne patients (43,44) (R. H. Brown, personal communication).

Neurofibromatosis

Neurofibromatosis is characterized by multiple tumors originating from Schwann cells and in peripheral nerves; it frequently is also associated with CNS tumors (neurofibromas, meningiomas, gliomas). It is inherited as an autosomal dominant disease. Two separable phenotypic patterns have been described with different genetic loci. The first, called neurofibromatosis type I (NFI) or von Recklinghausen's neurofibromatosis (VRNF) affects primarily the peripheral nervous system. The other form, NFII, affects the central nervous system, particularly the eighth cranial nerves. It is also called bilateral acoustic neurofibromatosis (BANF) (45). VRNF is one of the most common autosomal dominant conditions with an estimated prevalence of about one in 3,000; about half the cases represent new mutations. In addition to tumors on nerves, patients commonly demonstrate cutaneous pigmentary changes (café au lait spots) and iris hamartomas.

Recent linkage studies with anonymous and characterized probes have identified the gene for VRNF near the centromere on chromosome 17 (46,47). In 15 kindreds reported by Barker et al (46) no evidence of nonallelic heterogeneity was identified. In a second study of 13 additional families reported by Seizinger et al (47) linkage was shown to the locus of the nerve growth factor receptor gene on 17q12 17q22. However, crossovers that occurred with the latter locus indicate that a defect in the NFI gene is not in the nerve growth factor receptor gene itself.

Studies in NF type II show the disorder to be linked to chromosome 22 (48). In this condition, bilateral tumors occur on the eight cranial nerve, leading to deafness. The patients also exhibit a higher susceptibility to a variety of other nervous system tumors including meningiomas, gliomas, and neurofibromas of the spinal cord.

These discoveries have potential major implications for understanding tumor formation of CNS supporting cells (meningeal, astroglial, etc; see also the later section on brain tumors). Linked DNA markers will be particularly valuable in families with BANF for early identification and surgical treatment of the tumors.

Myotonic Dystrophy

Myotonic dystrophy (MD) is the most common form of adult-onset muscular dystrophy. It is a systemic disorder affecting the lens (cataracts), the heart (conduction defects), the skin and hair (frontal baldness), and, in some families, the brain (mental retardation). It is inherited as an autosomal dominant disorder. No documented cases of new mutation have been found. Several large families have been studied by linkage analysis, first with the use of apolipoprotein C2 (49) and, more recently, with anonymous DNA probes with informative RFLPs. Bartlett et al (50) examined six large MD families with probes selected from genomic DNA libraries enriched for chromosome 18. One clone, designated LDR152 (D19S19), was shown to be tightly linked to MD with a recombination fraction (θ) of 0.0 and a LOD score of 15.4. No crossover events were found in informative MD families when two different polymorphisms were used, which made the linkage of the probe to the gene locus exceedingly close. The MD locus resides on the q arm of the chromosome 19 near the centromere.

Familial Amyloidotic Polyneuropathy

Neurological abnormalities associated with amyloid deposition take several forms. The genetic basis of one of these, familial amyloidotic polyneuropathy (FAP), has been completely elucidated (51). FAP is an autosomal dominant disorder first described by Andrade in Portuguese families (52). Families of Jewish, Japanese, and Swedish lineage have also been identified. The disease has an onset in adults with symptoms and signs of distal extremity sensory loss and weakness. Autonomic nervous system involvement is prominent, with postural hypotension, anhidrosis, impotence, and gastrointestinal dysfunction. Symptoms often begin as early as the third decade, but in some pedigrees occur as late as the sixth or seventh decade. The disease results in the deposition of amyloid fibrils (β-pleated protein polymers) in peripheral nerve, heart, and kidneys, but not in the brain or other tissues of the central nervous system.

The disease in most pedigrees examined is caused by a single-base pair mutation on chromosome 18 of the gene that encodes for the protein transthyretin (formerly called prealbumin), a tetrameric 56-kD serum transport protein for thyroxine and vitamin A (retinoic acid). In Japanese, Portuguese, and Swedish families with FAP a single base pair change results in the substitution of methionine for valine at position 30 in transthyretin. A different base pair error causes substitution of phenylala-

TABLE 7.2. Protein variants associated with hereditary amyloidosis

Amyloid protein	Position	Mutation	Geographic location
Transthyretin	30	Val → Met	Portugal, Japan, Sweden, Italy, Greece, England, United States
Transthyretin	33	Phe → Ile	Israel
Transthyretin	60	Thr → Ala	West Virginia
Transthyretin	77	Ser → Tyr	Illinois (German extraction)
Transthyretin	84	Ile → Ser	Indiana (Swiss extraction)
Transthyretin	111	Leu → Met	Denmark

Reproduced from Benson and Wallace (51). Copyright 1989, McGraw-Hill, New York.

nine for isoleucine at position 33 in an Israeli pedigree; yet other substitutions have been found in other families (Table 7.2). These family studies of FAP strongly suggest that the mutation in transthyretin is both the genetic and the biochemical basis of the disease (53–56).

The gene for transthyretin has now been fully characterized. The nucleotide sequence of the gene spans 70 kb and consists of four exons and three introns.

An important unresolved question remains as to what mechanism or mechanisms might lead to the delayed onset of the disease until adulthood. Saraiva et al (57) examined this question in two Portuguese families, one with typical early-adult onset and the other with late-life onset. Plasma samples were analyzed for protein abnormalities in transthyretin. Leukocyte DNA, subjected to the restriction endonuclease, NsiI, was examined for RFLPs. In both early- and late-onset cases, and in presymptomatic children, the same quantitative abnormalities were found in transthyretin. Abnormal transthyretin (Met[30]) was shown to circulate in plasma early in life. It appears therefore, that the preclinical phase of the disease cannot be accounted for by developmental repression of the mutant gene, since the same genetic mutation was expressed early in life in both early- and late-onset cases. The factors that determine the rate of deposition of the abnormal protein as amyloid in tissues remain unknown. The protective mechanisms that delay onset of symptoms in one pedigree and not in another will be important to discern because of their implications for treatment.

CNS Tumors and Suppressor Oncogenes

Understanding cellular processes that determine normal cell differentiation and the termination of cell division are important for approaching mechanisms of tumor formation. Tumor development "may be viewed as the gradual emancipation of a clone of somatic cells from the complex controls that regulate its growth" (58). The genes that may influence the cellular growth adversely leading to tumor formation have been called oncogenes. A second type of gene, whose normal function appears to be the suppression of cellular division and growth is called an antioncogene or tumor suppressor gene.

The category of genes that can suppress tumor formation in nervous system tissue has received considerable experimental attention. Loss or mutational inactivation of "recessive cancer genes" is now speculated on good evidence to play a role in the formation of retinoblastoma, meningioma, acoustic neuromas, and hemangioblastoma (von Hippel-Lindau disease).

Retinoblastoma

Retinoblastoma is ordinarily a rare malignancy of childhood. Most cases are sporadic and unilateral. About 15% of cases, however, are inherited and occur bilaterally. Hereditary cases are transmitted phenotypically as an autosomal dominant trait. The locus for the tumor suppressor gene in retinoblastoma is chromosome 13q14; deletions of DNA in this region from both chromosomes are associated with tumor development. Inherited tumors occur when retinoblasts with one defective gene copy in this region due to a *germinal mutation* undergo a second *somatic mutational* or "second hit" of the chromosome carrying the normal allele, resulting in loss of the remaining normal copy of the gene. The defect leading to tumor formation appears to be the loss of both copies of a normal gene that regulates cell division and growth.

Cavenee and Dryja and co-workers (59,60) used DNA probes homologous to single-copy DNA sequences spaced along the q arm of chromosome 13 to compare RFLPs of DNA from tumor tissue with DNA derived from lymphocytes in the same patients in pedigrees with inherited retinoblastoma. Loss of the one normal gene that unmasks recessive mutation at the retinoblastoma locus was shown to occur by several different mechanisms, including nondisjunction, reduplication, mitotic recombination, gene conversion, or point mutation. Fung et al (61) found that 16 of 40 retinoblastomas probed with a cDNA to the retinoblastoma gene had identifiable structural changes, including in two cases homozygous internal deletions. It now seems likely that the "normal gene" that is mutant in retinoblastoma has been identified. Sequential cloning of adjacent DNA by chromosome walking led to isolation of a 70-kb portion of the human 13q14 fragment that hybridizes to RNA derived from human retinal cells and tumor (62). A 4.7-kb RNA transcript was identified, and it appears to correspond to the RNA found by Lee et al (63) that codes for a protein of 816 amino acids. Discerning the function of this protein, which appears to be a DNA-binding protein and is absent in retinoblastoma, will be important for understanding mechanisms of suppression of tumor growth.

Acoustic Neurofibromas

Similar strategies have been used to examine NFII. Seizinger and colleagues (64,65) examined tissue obtained from these tumors in search of chromosomal deletions that might provide a clue to the site of the chromosomal abnormality. DNA from patients with bilateral acoustic neuromas was compared with DNA from the patient's own leukocytes. Tumor tissue from these patients consistently demonstrated loss of a region of chromosome 22. These workers have subsequently produced a panel of DNA probes for chromosome 22 and have shown that families with NFII show linkage to chromosome 22, whereas families with NFI (VRNF), a disorder associated with peripheral neuromas, show negative linkage to chromosome 22 and positive linkage to chromosome 17. At this juncture it appears that the central form of the disease is analogous to retinoblastoma due to a "second-hit" mutation resulting in loss of a cell growth-controlling gene on chromosome 22. Precise definition of the genetic defects in these conditions remains to be accomplished, but this discovery will also have important implications for understanding growth characteristics of several central nervous system tumors.

Meningioma

Several reports, using molecular genetic approaches, have also shown a frequent association of DNA deletions on chromosome 22 in sporadic meningiomas (66,67).

Von Hippel-Lindau Disease

Von Hippel-Lindau disease is an autosomal dominant disorder with inherited susceptibility to various forms of cancer, including hemangio-blastomas of the CNS, pheochromocytomas, and renal cell carcinoma. Using the clue that renal cell carcinomas have been associated with deletion of portions of chromosome 3p, Seizinger and colleagues (68) examined nine families with von Hippel-Lindau disease and found that the disease was linked to the human homolog of the RAF oncogene, which maps to chromosome 3p25. They speculate that similar mechanisms of tumor suppression may be associated with both the inherited and sporadic forms of the disease (ie, that a recessive oncogene or tumor suppressor gene, when deleted from both chromosomes leads to tumor growth).

Molecular Genetic Approaches to Neuropsychiatric Diseases

The strategies of linkage analysis have used one of four techniques: the random marker approach, the candidate gene approach, the candidate chromosome approach, and the tumor deletion approach.

Random Marker Approach

Several examples cited above indicate the power of using pedigree linkage analysis with DNA probes showing RFLPs to locate the chromosomal locus of the diseases. Several groups of investigators are systematically developing probes that span the entire human genome. Already more than 95% is covered by such probes. The total number of equally spaced probes required is estimated to be between 200 and 500. If one estimates that probes spaced at 10 cM (approximately 10,000,000 base pairs) are sufficiently close to detect linkage, then

$$\frac{3 \times 10^9 \text{ bp}}{1 \times 10^7 \text{ bp}} = 300$$

probes are required to span the entire genome at 10cM spaces.

The use of the random marker approach, first successful in HD, now promises to also be successful in many other diseases such as familial spastic paraparesis, familial amyotrophic lateral sclerosis, and in torsion dystonia of autosomal dominant form. What of those psychiatric disorders concerning which current evidence supports inheritance as a major factor (ie, manic-depressive illness, schizophrenia, drug addiction, alcoholism)? The essential ingredient for successful study is the acquisition of a *large* pedigree in which *inheritance is established and where phenotypic expression of the disorder is sufficiently reliable to make clinical diagnosis unequivocal.* If not, determination of linkage can be subject to error—either concluding positive linkage when it is not present or a negative linkage when it is present.

The difficulties encountered so far in ascertaining the locus of inheritance in manic-depressive disease is particularly informative. Several linkage studies have now been reported encouraged by the growing clinical evidence that individuals in some families are genetically predisposed to manic-depressive illness. The first clue to the chromosomal location of one such gene came from studies in the Old Order Amish of Pennsylvania (69). Recent evidence from this group suggested that RFLPs from two genes on chromosome 11p are frequently linked with the affective disorder (70). Manic-depressive disorder linked to chromosome 11 is of considerable interest because the marker genes on that chromosome are close to the gene-encoding tyrosine hydroxylase, the rate-limiting enzyme for the biosynthesis of the catecholamines. Abnormalities of catecholamine function have long been considered a potential pathogenetic mechanism in manic-depressive illness. However, two other groups of investigators have shown in six other families, three from Iceland and three from North America, that linkage with the same probes to chromosome 11 gave negative log of the odds (LOD) scores (71,72). These findings indicate the possibility of either nonallelic genetic heterogeneity for manic-depressive illness or of an error in the analysis of the Amish pedigree. Baron et al (73) studying pedigrees of patients in Israel, and Mendlewicz et al (74) examining patients in Belgium, both demonstrated genetic linkage between bipolar affective illness and the X chromosome. An interesting association between the X linkage and color blindness was noted in these families. These data, taken as a whole, suggest that manic-depressive illness, which in some families takes primarily a bipolar form, and in others is unipolar, is caused by several *different* disorders.

It is unclear whether families with schizophrenia will present a similar opportunity for genetic linkage. Several studies are in progress. Genetic linkage analysis will likely be most difficult for traits like propensity to alcoholism or drug addiction. Unless biochemical parameters are established to detect susceptibility, it seems difficult to imagine that clinical diagnosis alone will be sufficiently reliable to achieve significant results in a statistical linkage study.

Candidate Gene Approach

As reviewed recently by McKusick (75), there are at least three variations of this approach. The first is based on the question: Does the disorder map to the same chromosomal locus as the candidate gene? An example is Wilson's disease, in connection with which the question has been asked: Is the primary genetic defect in the structural gene for ceruloplasmin? In this case the answer is no, because the disease gene maps to 13q and the candidate gene to 3q. In this case, this experimental approach has permitted exclusion of one possible cause of the disease. In another example, Pelizaeus-Merzbacher disease, a neurologic disease that causes degeneration in cerebral white matter, and which is known to be X-linked, a candidate gene encoding for a lipid-myelin proteolipid protein was shown to be abnormal in some patients, thereby placing the genetic locus at Xq22.

A second candidate gene approach uses RFLPs to a known gene, which shows no recombination to the disease locus in families. This approach is not without limitations, however, because a RFLP locus close to a gene may show recombination so infrequently as to be missed at first. Such a circumstance appeared in our experience with the C4H probe in HD. Although initial observations showed no recombination in three extended families (17), subsequent studies have revealed recombinations (J. Gusella, unpublished).

A third candidate gene approach involves display of a suspect gene by Southern blot analysis to examine for abnormalities of size in DNA fragments. This approach has limitations, however, since failure to find abnormalities does not exclude the candidate gene as a cause; in Lesch-Nyhan disease and in Duchenne dystrophy, for example, more than 50% of cases fail to show any abnormality, presumably because the mutation is so subtle—a single base pair change, for example.

Candidate Chromosomal Approach

Using this approach, a particular chromosome is studied in detail. In FAD, the clue was the neuropathologic changes occurring in trisomy 21 (Down's syndrome) which resemble AD. This led to detailed examination of chromosome 21 with informative probes. The search was successful.

Tumor Deletion Approach

Using knowledge of the association between chromosomal deletions on 3p and renal cell carcinoma, and the increased frequency of this same tumor in von Hippel-Lindau disease, led to the successful linkage in nine families of this disorder to RFLPs from markers on 3p (68). Similar observations of deletions of chromosome 22 in meningiomas (66,67) with deletions in acoustic neuroma led to the successful linkage to chromosome 22 for NFII.

Looking to the Future

Recent applications of molecular biology have yielded important new insights into diseases of the CNS. The structure and function of several genes causing neurological disorders are currently being defined. Information already available shows that the molecular changes underlying the phenotypic expression of a given disease can encompass a range of genetic errors. The modifying factors that determine variations in the phenotypic expression of a single genetic abnormality—for example, what factors determine early versus late onset of the illness in different individuals—remain essentially undefined.

What are the future implications of these discoveries for neurology and psychiatry? First, linkage analysis with RFLPs can now be applied to many of the other genetic disorders provided families with adequately defined expression of the disease are available for study. Second, linkage analysis can now be used for genetic counseling in HD, MD, DMD, and in those families with FAD where linkage has been documented. Third, improved strategies for cloning large segments of DNA, as recently shown in yeast, and methods to separate segments on gel electrophoresis should speed the development of physical linkage maps to locate, define, and clone abnormal genes. A fourth issue may be the most challenging: how to discover the functions of genes that are structurally characterized. It will likely be a complex undertaking, after discovery of a protein abnormality, to identify its normal function. One promising approach will be to introduce abnormal genes into transgenic animals and to examine them for phenotypic expression of the disease. Animal models of disease have already been of great value in several autosomal recessive diseases of the CNS.

The possibility of gene therapy for disorders affecting the central
nervous system seems remote. Partial correction of the gene defect in the
shiverer mouse has been accomplished in transgenic experiments (76).
Development of viral vectors specific for individual cell types is the
subject of current research in many laboratories. At present, one can be
optimistic that genes can be introduced into replicating cells with these
techniques, but whether *in vivo* site-specific gene insertion will be
possible into postmitotic brain neurons remains to be shown.

Acknowledgments. Portions of this review are reproduced with permission from an earlier article by the author that appeared in *Science*.

References

1. O'Brien JS (1983). The metabolic basis of inherited disease. In JB Stanbury,
   J Wyngaarden, DS Fredrickson, JL Goldstein, MS Brown eds. McGraw-Hill,
   New York, pp 94–969.
2. Myerowitz R, Piekarz R, Neufeld EF, Shows TB, Suzuki K (1985). Human
   beta-hexosaminidase alpha chain: Coding sequence and homology with beta
   chain. *Proc National Acad Sci USA* 82:7830–7834.
3. Proia RL (1988). Gene encoding the human β-hexosaminidase β-chain:
   Extensive homology of intron placement in the α- and β-chain genes. *Proc
   National Acad Sci USA* 85:1883–1887.
4. Tsuji S, Choudary PV, Martin BM, Stubblefield BK et al (1987). A mutation in
   the human glucocerebrosidase gene in neuronopathic Gaucher's disease.
   N Engl J Med 316:570–575.
5. Botstein D, White RL, Skolnick M, Davis RW (1980). Construction of a
   genetic linkage map in man using restriction fragment length polymorphisms.
   Am J Hum Genet 32:314–331.
6. Housman D, Gusella JF (1981). Use of recombinant DNA techniques for
   linkage studies in genetically based neurological disorders. In ES Gershon,
   S Matthysse, XO Breakfield, RD Ciaranello, eds. Boxwood Press 1981;
   p 17–24.
7. Gusella JF, Tanzi RE, Anderson MA (1984). DNA markers for nervous
   system diseases. *Science* 225:1320–1326.
8. Gusella JF (1986). DNA polymorphism and human disease. *Ann Rev Biochem*
   55:831–854.
9. Martin JB (1984). Huntington's disease: New approaches to an old problem.
   Neurology 34:1059–1067.
10. Martin JB, Gusella JF (1986). Huntington's disease: pathogenesis and man-
    agement. *N Engl J Med* 316:1018–1020.
11. Kowall N, Ferrante R, Martin JB (1987). Patterns of cell loss in Huntington's
    disease. *Trends Neurosci* 10:24–29.
12. Beal, MF, Kowal NW, Ellison DW, Mazurek MF, et al (1986). Replication of
    the neurochemical characteristics of Huntington's disease by quinolinic acid.
    Nature (London) 321:168–171.
13. Marx JL (1987). Animals yield clues to Huntington's disease. *Science*
    238:1510–1511.

14. Gusella JF, Wexler NS, Conneally PM, Naylor SL, et al (1983). A polymorphic DNA marker genetically linked to Huntington's disease. *Nature (London)* 306:234–238.
15. Gusella JF (1986). Molecular genetics of Huntington's disease. *Cold Spring Harbor Symp Quant Biol* 51:359–364.
16. Blanche H, Zunec R, Gilliam C, Hartley D, et al (1987). A human anonymous low copy number clone, 4c11 (D6S4), localized to 6p12-6p21, detects 2 RFLPs, one of which is moderately polymorphic. *Nucleic Acids Res* 15:5902–5905.
17. Gilliam TC, Bucan M, MacDonald ME, Zimmer M, et al (1987). A DNA segment encoding two genes very tightly linked to Huntington's disease. *Science* 238:950–952.
18. Wexler NS, Young AB, Tanzi RE, Travers H, et al (1987). Homozygotes for Huntington's disease. *Nature (London)* 326:194–197.
19. Meissen GJ, Myers RH, Mastromauro CA (1988). Predictive testing for Huntington's disease with use of a linked DNA marker. *N Engl J Med* 318:535–542.
20. Katzman R (1986). Alzheimer's disease. *N Engl J Med* 314:964–969.
21. Tanzi RE, St George-Hyslop PH, Haines JL, Polinsky RJ, et al (1987). The genetic defect in familial Alzheimer's disease in not tightly linked to the amyloid beta-protein gene. *Nature (London)* 329:156–157.
22. Glenner GG, Wong CW (1984). Alzheimer's disease: Initial report of the purification and characterization of a novel cerebrovascular amyloid protein. *Biochem Biophys Res Commun* 120:885–890.
23. Masters CL, Simms G, Weinman NA, Multhaup G, McDonald BL, Beyreuther K, et al (1985). Amyloid plaque core protein in Alzheimer's disease and Down syndrome. *Proc National Acad Sci USA* 82:4245–4249.
24. Robakis NK, Wisniewski HM, Jenkins EC, Devine-Gage EA, et al (1987). Chromosome 21q21 sublocalisation of gene encoding beta-amyloid peptide incerebral vessels and neuritic (senile) plaques of people with Alzheimer disease and Down syndrome [letter] *Lancet* 1:384–385.
25. Goldgaber D, Lerman MI, McBride OW, Saffiotti U, Gajdusek DC (1987). Characterization and chromosomal localization of a cDNA encoding brain amyloid of Alzheimer's disease. *Science* 235:877–800.
26. Kang J, Lemaire HG, Unterbeck A, Salbaum JM, et al (1987). The precursor of Alzheimer's disease amyloid A4 protein resembles a cell surface receptor. *Nature (London)* 325:733–736.
27. Tanzi RE, Gusella JF, Watkins PC, Bruns GA, et al (1987). Amyloid beta protein gene: cDNA, mRNA distribution, and genetic linkage near the Alzheimer locus. *Science* 235:880–884.
28. Delabar JM, Goldgaber D, Lamour Y, Nicle A, et al (1987). Beta amyloid gene duplication in Alzheimer's disease and karyotypically normal Down syndrome. *Science* 235:1390–1392.
29. St. George-Hyslop PH, Tanzi RE, Polinsky TJ et al (1987). Absence of duplication of chromosome 21 genes in familial and sporadic Alzheimer's disease. *Science* 238:664–669.
30. Tanzi RE, Bird ED, Latt SA, Neve RL (1987). The amyloid β-protein gene is not duplicated in brains from patients with Alzheimer's disease. *Science* 238:666–668.

31. Podlisny MB, Lee G, Selkoe DJ (1987). Gene dosage of the amyloid beta precursor protein in Alzheimer's disease. *Science* 238:669–671.
32. Bahmanyar S, Higgins GA, Goldgaber D, Lewis DA, et al (1987). Localization of amyloid beta protein messenger RNA in brains from patients with Alzheimer's disease. *Science* 237:77–80.
33. Ponte P, Gonzalez-DeWhitt P, Schilling J, Miller J, et al (1988). A new A4 amyloid mRNA contains a domain homologous to serine proteinase inhibitors. *Nature (London)* 331:525–527.
34. Tanzi RE, McClatchey AI, Lamperti ED, Villa-Komaroff L, et al (1988). Protease inhibitor domain encoded by an amyloid protein precursor mRNA associated with Alzheimer's disease. *Nature (London)* 331:528–530.
35. Brooke MH, Fenichel GM, Griggs RC, Mendell JR, et al (1983). Clinical investigation in Duchenne dystrophy: 2. Determination of the "power" of therapeutic trials based on the natural history. *Muscle Nerve* 6:91–103.
36. Ray PN, Belfall B, Duff C, et al (1985). Cloning of the breakpoint of an xp21 translocation associated with Duchenne muscular dystrophy. *Nature (London)* 318:672–675.
37. van Ommen GJ, Verkerk JM, Hofker MH, Monaco AP, et al (1986). A physical map of 4 million bp around the Duchenne muscular dystrophy gene on the human X-chromosome. *Cell* 47:499–504.
38. Burmeister M, Lehrach H (1986). Long-range restriction map around the Duchenne muscular dystrophy gene. *Nature (London)* 324:582.
39. Monaco AP, Neve RL, Colletti-Feener C, et al (1986). Isolation of candidate cDNAs for portions of the Duchenne muscular dystrophy gene. *Nature (London)* 323:646–650.
40. Monaco AP, Bertelson CH, Coletti-Feener C, Kunkel LM (1987). Localization and cloning of xp21 deletion breakpoints involved in muscular dystrophy. *Hum Genet* 75:221–227.
41. Koenig M, Hoffman EP, Bertelson CJ, et al (1987). Complete cloning of the Duchenne muscular dystrophy (DMD) cDNA and preliminary genomic organization of the DMD gene in normal and affected individuals. *Cell* 50:509–517.
42. Hoffman EP, Monaco AP, Feener CC, Kunkel M (1987). Conservation of the Duchenne muscular dystrophy gene in mice and humans. *Science* 238: 347–349.
43. Hoffman EP, Brown RH, Kunkel LM (1987). Dystrophin: The protein product of the Duchenne muscular dystrophy locus. *Cell* 51:919–928.
44. Hoffman EP, Knudson CM, Campbell KP, Kunkel LM (1987). Subcellular fractionation of dystrophin to the trials of skeletal muscle. *Nature (London)* 330:754–757.
45. Martuza RL, Seizinger BR, Jacoby LB, Rouleau GA, Gusella, JF (1988). The molecular biology of human glial tumors. *Trends Neurosci* 11:22–27.
46. Barker D, Wright E, Nguyen K, Cannon L, et al (1987). Gene for von Recklinghausen neurofibromatosis is in the pericentromeric region of chromosome 17. *Science* 236:1100–1102.
47. Seizinger BR, Rouleau GA, Ozelius LJ, Lane AH, et al (1987). Genetic linkage of von Recklinghausen neurofibromatosis to the nerve growth factor receptor gene. *Cell* 49:589–594.
48. Martuza RL, Eldridge R (1988). Neurofibromatosis 2. *N Engl J Med* 318: 684–687.

49. Pericak-Vance MA, et al (1986). Tight linkage of apolipoprotein C2 to myotonic dystrophy on chromosome. *Neurology* 36:1418.
50. Bartlett RJ, et al (1987). A new probe for the diagnosis of myotonic muscular dystrophy. *Science* 236:1100–1103.
51. Benson MD, Wallace MR (1989). Familial amyloidotic polyneuropathy. In CR Scriver, AL Beaudet, WS Sly, D Valle, *The Metabolic Basis of Inherited Disease*, Sixth Edition. McGraw-Hill, New York, pp 3647–3681.
52. Andrade C (1986). A peculiar form of peripheral neuropathy: Familial atypical generalized amyloids with special involvement of the peripheral nerves. *Brain* 75:408–413.
53. Wallace MR, Dwulet FE, Williams EC, Conneally PM, Benson MD (1988). Identification of a new hereditary amyloidosis prealbumin variant, Tyr-77, and detection of the gene by DNA analysis. *J Clin Invest* 81:189–193.
54. Maeda S, Mita S, Araki S, Shimada K (1986). Structure and expression of the mutant prealbumin gene associated with familial amyloidotic polyneuropathy. *Mol Biol Med* 3:329–338.
55. Yoshioka K, Sasaki H, Yoshioka N, Furuya H, et al (1986). Structure of the mutant prealbumin gene responsible for familial amyloidotic polyneuropathy. *Mol Biol Med* 3:319–328.
56. Whitehead AS, et al (1984). Cloning of human prealbumin complementary DNA. Localization of the gene to chromosome 18 and detection of a variant prealbumin allele in a family with familial amyloid polyneuropathy. *Mol Biol Med* 2:411–423.
57. Saraiva MJM, Costra PP, Goodman DS (1986). Genetic expression of a transthyretin mutation in typical and late onset Portuguese families with familial amyloidotic polyneuropathy. *Neurology* 36:1413–1415.
58. Klein G (1987). The approaching era of the tumor suppressor genes. *Science* 238:1539–1545.
59. Cavenee WK, Murphree AL, Shull MM, Benedict WF, et al 91986). Prediction of familial predisposition to retinoblastoma. *N Engl J Med* 314:1201–1207.
60. Dryja TP, Rapaport JM, Epstein J, Goorin Am, et al (1984). Homozygosity of chromosome 13 in retinoblastoma. *N Engl J Med* 310:550–553.
61. Fung Y-KT, Murphree AL, T'ang A, et al (1987). Structural evidence for the authenticity of the human retinoblastoma gene. *Science* 236:1657–1661.
62. Friend SH, Bernards R, Rogelj S, Weinberg RA, et al (1986). A human DNA segment with properties of the gene that predisposes to retinoblastoma and osteosarcoma. *Nature (London)* 323:643.
63. Lee WH, Bookstein R, Hong F, Young LJ, et al (1987). Human retinoblastoma susceptibility gene: cloning, identification, and sequence. *Science* 235:1394–1399.
64. Seizinger BR, Martuza RL, Gusella JF (1986). Loss of genes on chromosome 22 in tumorigenesis of human acoustic neuroma. *Nature (London)* 322:644.
65. Seizinger BR, Rouleau G, Ozelius LJ, Lane AH, et al (1987). Common pathogenetic mechanism for three tumor types in bilateral acoustic neurofibromatosis. *Science* 236:317–319.
66. Dumanski JP, Carlbom E, Collins VP, Nordenskjold M. (1987). Deletion mapping of a locus on human chromosome 22 involved in the oncogenesis of meningioma. *Proc National Acad Sci USA* 84:9275–9279.

67. Seizinger BR, Tanzi RE, Gilliam TC, Bader JL, et al (1988). Genetic linkage analysis of neurofibromatosis with DNA markers. *Ann NY Acad Sci* 486: 304–310.
68. Seizinger BR, Rouleau GA, Ozelius LJ, Lane AH, et al (1988). Von Hippel-Lindau disease maps to the region of chromosome 3 associated with renal cell carcinoma. *Nature (London)* 332:268–269.
69. Graham GJ, Hall TJ, Cummings MR (1984). Isolation of repetitive DNA sequences from human chromosome 21. *Am J Hum Genet* 36:25–35.
70. Egeland JA, Gerhard DS, Pauls DL, Sussex JN, et al (1987). Bipolar affective disorders linked to DNA markers on chromosome 11. *Nature (London)* 325:783–787.
71. Hodgkinson S, Sherrington R, Gurling H, Marchbanks R, et al (1987). Molecular genetic evidence for heterogeneity in manic depression. *Nature (London)* 325:805–806.
72. Detera-Wadleigh SD, Berrettini WH, Goldin LR, Boorman D, et al (1987). Close linkage of c-Harvey-ras-1 and the insulin gene to affective disorder is ruled out in three North American pedigrees. *Nature (London)* 325:806–808.
73. Baron M, Risch N, Hamburger R, Mandel B, et al (1987). Genetic linkage between X-chromosome markers and bipolar affective illness. *Nature (London)* 326:289–292.
74. Medlewicz J, Simon P, Sevy S, Charon F, et al (1987). Polymorphic DNA market on X chromosome and manic depression. *Lancet* 1:1230–1232.
75. McKusick V (1988). The morbid anatomy of the human genome: A review of the gene mapping in clinical medicine. *Medicine* 67:1–19.
76. Readhead C, Popko B, Takahashi N, Shine HD, et al (1987). Expression of a myelin basic protein gene in transgenic shiverer mice: correction of the dysmyelinating phenotype. *Cell* 48:703–712.

Index

Note: Page numbers in *italics* refer to illustrations; page numbers followed by t refer to tables.